Robotic Surgery

Guest Editor

JOHN ZENDER, RN, BS, CNOR

PERIOPERATIVE NURSING CLINICS

www.periopnursing.theclinics.com

Consulting Editor
NANCY GIRARD, PhD, RN, FAAN

September 2011 • Volume 6 • Number 3

SAUNDERS an imprint of ELSEVIER, Inc.

W.B. SAUNDERS COMPANY
A Division of Elsevier Inc.

1600 John F. Kennedy Boulevard • Suite 1800 • Philadelphia, Pennsylvania 19103-2899

http://www.periopnursing.theclinics.com

PERIOPERATIVE NURSING CLINICS Volume 6, Number 3
September 2011 ISSN 1556-7931, ISBN-13: 978-1-4557-0486-6

Editor: Katie Hartner
Developmental Editor: Donald Mumford

Perioperative Nursing Clinics (ISSN 1556-7931) is published quarterly by Elsevier, 360 Park Avenue South, New York, NY 10010. Months of issue are March, June, September and December. Business and Editorial Offices: 1600 John F. Kennedy Blvd., Suite 1800, Philadelphia, PA 19103-2899. Customer Service Office: 11830 Westline Industrial Drive, St. Louis, MO 63146. Periodicals postage paid at New York, NY and at additional mailing offices. Subscription prices are $124.00 per year (domestic individuals), $213.00 per year (domestic institutions), $61.00.00 per year (domestic students/ residents), $161.00 per year (international individuals), $245.00 per year (international institutions), and $65.00 per year (International students/residents). Foreign air speed delivery is included in all *Clinics* subscription prices. All prices are subject to change without notice. **POSTMASTER:** Send change of address to *Perioperative Nursing Clinics*, Customer Service (orders, claims, online, change of address): Elsevier Periodicals Customer Service, 11830 Westline Industrial Drive, St. Louis, MO 63146. Tel: 1-800-654-2452 (U.S. and Canada). Fax: 314-523-5170. E-mail: journalscustomerservice-usa@elsevier.com (for print support); journalsonlinesupport-usa@elsevier.com (for online support).

Reprints. For copies of 100 or more, of articles in this publication, please contact the Commercial Rights Department, Elsevier Inc., 360 Park Avenue South, New York, NY 10010-1710; Phone: (+1) 212-633-3813; Fax: (+1) 212-462-1935; E-mail: reprints@elsevier.com.

Printed and bound by CPI Group (UK) Ltd, Croydon, CR0 4YY
Transferred to Digital Print 2012

Contributors

CONSULTING EDITOR

NANCY GIRARD, PhD, RN, FAAN
Nurse Collaborations, Boerne, Texas; Clinical Associate Professor, Acute Nursing Care Department, University of Texas Health Science Center, San Antonio, Texas

GUEST EDITOR

JOHN ZENDER, RN, BS, CNOR
Surgical Services, St Joseph's Medical Center, Brainerd, Minnesota

AUTHORS

FLORIAN AUGUSTIN, MD
Department of Visceral, Transplant and Thoracic Surgery, Innsbruck Medical University, Innsbruck, Austria

DAVID L. BARTLETT, MD
Bernard Fisher Professor of Surgery and Chief, Division of Surgical Oncology, Department of Surgery, University of Pittsburgh Medical Center Cancer Pavilion, Pittsburgh, Pennsylvania

JOHANNES BODNER, MD, MSc, FETCS
Chief, Division of Surgery, Department of General, Visceral, Thoracic, Transplant and Pediatric Surgery, University Hospital Giessen and Marburg, Giessen, Germany

MARIANA BOYLE, RN, BSN, CNOR
Clinical Perioperative Nurse Educator, University of Chicago Medical Center, Chicago, Illinois

DAVID S. CHOU, MD, FACS
Pacific Urology, Inc, Honolulu, Hawaii

DAVID A. GELLER, MD, FACS
Richard L. Simmons Professor of Surgery; Department of Surgery, Starzl Transplant Institute; Co-Director, UPMC Liver Cancer Center, University of Pittsburgh, Pittsburgh, Pennsylvania

RAJ K. GOEL, MD, FRCSC
Clinical Fellow, Glickman Urological and Kidney Institute, Cleveland Clinic Foundation, Cleveland, Ohio

KAMRAN IDREES, MD
Surgical Oncology Fellow, Division of Surgical Oncology, Department of Surgery, University of Pittsburgh Medical Center Cancer Pavilion, Pittsburgh, Pennsylvania

JIHAD H. KAOUK, MD
Director, Center for Advanced Laparoscopic and Robotic Surgery, Glickman Urological and Kidney Institute, Cleveland Clinic Foundation, Cleveland, Ohio

PHILLIP MUCKSAVAGE, MD
University of California Irvine Medical Center, Orange, California

KEVIN TRI NGUYEN, MD, PhD
Department of Surgery, Starzl Transplant Institute, UPMC Liver Cancer Center, University of Pittsburgh, Pittsburgh, Pennsylvania

GERALD Y. TAN, MBChB, MRCSEd, MMed, FAMS
Ferdinand C. Valentine Fellow, Brady Foundation Department of Urology, Weill Medical College of Cornell University; Clinical Fellow, Lefrak Institute of Robotic Surgery, New York Presbyterian Hospital, New York, New York; and Associate Consultant, Department of Urology, Tan Tock Seng Hospital, Singapore

ASHUTOSH K. TEWARI, MD, MCh
Ronald P. Lynch Associate Professor of Urologic Oncology, Brady Foundation Department of Urology, Weill Medical College of Cornell University; and Director, Lefrak Institute of Robotic Surgery, New York Presbyterian Hospital, New York, New York

CHRISTINA G. THELL, RN, BS, CNOR
Surgical Services, St Joseph's Medical Center, Brainerd, Minnesota

CYNTHIA C. THOMAS, BSN, RN, CNOR
Endoscopy Resource Nurse, Robotic Coordinator, Woman's Hospital, Baton Rouge, Louisiana

RENA THOMPSON, RN, MSN, CNS-BC
Clinical Perioperative Nurse Educator, University of Chicago Medical Center, Chicago, Illinois

ANNEMARIE WEISSENBACHER, MD
Department of Visceral, Transplant and Thoracic Surgery, Innsbruck Medical University, Innsbruck, Austria

JOHN ZENDER, RN, BS, CNOR
Surgical Services, St Joseph's Medical Center, Brainerd, Minnesota

Contents

Keeping Pace with Robotic Technology 201

Rena Thompson and Mariana Boyle

> Robotic surgery has recently changed the face of surgery, and robotic technology has been in constant fluctuation over the last 10 years. The University of Chicago Medical Center (UCMC) originally purchased the Standard Robot da Vinci System during the early 2000s. Since then, we have purchased two additional da Vinci robot systems and discovered that each was an upgrade of the previous system. With each upgrade, the robotic trained staff's skills reverted from proficient/expert to novice. This article gives an overview of the robotic training and education program at UCMC and recommendations for future training and education.

Developing a Successful Robotic Surgery Program in a Rural Hospital 213

John Zender and Christina G. Thell

> Robotic surgery has become a standard in many large hospitals across the United States and the world. The surgical robot offers the surgeon a 3-dimensional view and increased dexterity in addition to providing the benefits of laparoscopic surgery to the patient (eg, shorter hospital stays, decreased pain, fewer postoperative complications). The next progression for robotic surgery is a move to rural venues. For many small, rural hospitals, however, obtaining a robot may be cost prohibitive, and these facilities may need to explore sources of funding for the program. Developing a robotics program requires intense training by surgeons and all surgical team members. Effective marketing of the program and the dedication and hard work of surgical team members and administrators are vital to ensure the success of the program.

The ability to help shape the future is a rewarding opportunity for the perioperative nurse ready for a challenge. Robotics has given perioperative nurses the opportunity to adapt their practice, think creatively, and develop efficient clinical practices to care for their patient's safety. The prospect of developing a robotic surgery program can be quite overwhelming. Using the skills and knowledge of an experienced perioperative nurse will allow development of an efficient robotic program.

The defining characteristic of perioperative nursing is patient advocacy— our foundation of practice. Although we are inundated with technology, new procedures, coordinating staff, and financial concerns, patient advocacy is at the forefront of what we do every day. With all the hype of robotic surgery, we must not forget our patients' perceptions of this new technology. It is our duty to counsel and comfort them as this new generation of robotic surgery sweeps the globe. This article discusses the role of patient advocate in perioperative nursing, patient percep- tions related to robotic surgery, and combining patient advocacy with robotic surgery.

Since the introduction of the da Vinci surgical system, urology has been at the forefront in the development and utilization of robotic surgery. Most radical prostatectomies are now performed using robotic assistance, while robotic assistance for renal surgery is rapidly increasing. In this review, the uses of the robot in urology, with a particular focus on the robot-assisted laparoscopic radical prostatectomies, will be examined.

Although minimally invasive hepatic resection surgery has shown decreased morbidity in select patients, conventional laparoscopic liver resection has inherent limitations with reduced freedom of movement within the abdominal cavity and 2-dimensional view of the operative field. Robotic liver surgery allows surgeons to perform advanced proce- dures with a potential for improved precision and ergonomics as well as a 3-dimensional view of the surgical site. However, use of the robot entails a steep learning curve and additional equipment. The purpose of this article is to summarize the emerging field of robotic liver surgery and include the authors' early experience with these operations.

In this article, the authors describe the evolution of urologic robotic systems and the current state-of-the-art features and existing limitations of the da Vinci S HD System (Intuitive Surgical, Inc). They then review promising innovations in scaling down the footprint of robotic platforms, the early experience with mobile miniaturized in vivo robots, advances in endoscopic navigation systems using augmented reality technologies and tracking devices, the emergence of technologies for robotic natural orifice transluminal endoscopic surgery and single-port surgery, advances in flexible robotics and haptics, the development of new virtual reality simulator training platforms compatible with the existing da Vinci system, and recent experiences with remote robotic surgery and telestration.

Several different mediastinal procedures for benign and malignant diseases have been proved to be feasible and safe when performed by a robotic minimally invasive approach. This article reviews the published data on robotic mediastinal surgery, focusing on technical aspects and perioperative outcomes. These are evaluated for differences and potential benefits over open and conventional minimally invasive techniques. Is there a need for the robot in the mediastinum? Is its application justified?

An increasing number of studies are reporting the outcomes and benefits of laparoscopic liver resection. This article reviews the literature with emphasis on a recent consensus conference on laparoscopic liver resection in 2008, the learning curve for laparoscopic liver surgery, laparoscopic major hepatectomies, oncologic outcomes of laparoscopic liver resection for hepatocellular carcinoma and colorectal cancer liver metastases, and the comparative benefits of laparoscopic versus open liver resection. Current evidence suggests that minimally invasive hepatic resection is safe and feasible with short-term benefits, no economic disadvantage, and no compromise to oncologic principles.

THE CLINICS ARE NOW AVAILABLE ONLINE!

Access your subscription at:
www.theclinics.com

Foreword

Robotics: Not Your Grandmother's Surgery

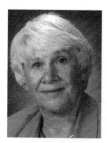

Nancy Girard, PhD, RN, FAAN
Consulting Editor

When my grandmother's generation had surgery, it was controlled and careful but it required a very invasive intrusion into the body. Incisions were sometimes huge and the recovery took weeks or even months. Hospitalization was most often required. The patient usually had considerable pain postoperatively, was more prone to wound infections, and ended up with very large scars. Recovery mainly depended upon the skills of the surgeon and his or her ability to be steady and meticulous in technique.

Today, the use of robots is changing the process of surgery. Robotic surgery allows for much smaller incisions (often just a puncture wound), less infection, less pain, and much shorter recovery time. While the surgeon is still the driver, the use of robotic instrumentation allows for greater precision, steadier instruments, and less invasive procedures. The patient most often has this type of surgery done in an ambulatory surgical center, meaning no hospitalization at all. Perioperative nurses must update their skill sets to work with the new technology, but the roles of patient advocate and maintainer of safety and the operating room environment remain staples in nursing.

The concept of machines doing repetitive labor has been around for centuries. Cesibius, a Greek inventor, made water clocks with movable figures as early as 270. Leonardo da Vinci designed a mechanical man in 1495 (and today's major surgical robotic system reflects his name). The most famous and scary artificial life idea was created by Mary Shelley in 1818 with her story about "Frankenstein." More recently, a science fiction writer who influenced technological developments was Isaac Asimov, who first used the word "robotics" to describe the development of robots and predicted the rise of a powerful robot industry.[1] While there are safety requirements

Perioperative Nursing Clinics 6 (2011) ix–x
doi:10.1016/j.cpen.2011.06.006
1556-7931/11/$ – see front matter

today for industrial robots, they are voluntary, not laws. Asimov's Robotic Laws are still unofficially considered to be pertinent. They are as follows:

- **LAW ZERO:** A robot may not injure humanity, or, through inaction, allow humanity to come to harm.
- **LAW ONE:** A robot may not injure a human being, or, through inaction, allow a human being to come to harm, unless this would violate a higher order law.
- **LAW TWO:** A robot must obey orders given it by human beings, except where such orders would conflict with a higher order law.
- **LAW THREE:** A robot must protect its own existence as long as such protection does not conflict with a higher order law.[2]

This issue of *Perioperative Nursing Clinics* presents "Robotic Surgery," with a wide variety of articles from specific surgical procedures to technology to patient care. While these surgeries may be increasing at many hospitals, the potential future possibilities are astounding and at times frightening. Only some of the robotic surgeries can be covered in this issue, but the broad use of robotics is expanding yearly. Robots are assisting in heart, brain, liver, lung, and prostate surgeries, as well as transplant surgeries. Care at a distance is also being implemented in areas that are without surgical care. For example, if there is a robot available on a battlefield, surgeons can repair damage immediately.

New information and technology continue to advance at a fast pace as better and more easily used discoveries evolve. For example, a robotic Leech used at Carnegie Mellon University's HeartLander, can inject drugs, heal hearts, and connect pacemakers. It is also engineered to destroy damaged tissue. The first tiny mobile robots (bots) to successfully navigate the frontal surface of a beating heart recently began journeying to the back of the heart to give physicians a total view of the heart.[3] Other items coming in the future definitely reflect science fiction: molecular "worms" that snake through your body and repair tissue, deliver drugs specifically for the individual at a target site, or rearrange damaged DNA. If we would publish another issue on robotic medicine and surgery in 10 years, it might be totally different than articles today. In fact, in the future the information in this issue might seem as basic as surgery decades ago appears today. The articles in this issue, however, present the newest information available today about robotic surgery that hopefully will assist everyone on the health care team. Thank goodness we live in an age where surgery now is not your grandmother's surgery, but I STILL have a perioperative nurse at my side if I need it.

Nancy Girard, PhD, RN, FAAN
Nurse Collaborations
8910 Buckskin Drive
Boerne, TX 78006-5565, USA

E-mail address:
ngirard2@satx.rr.com

REFERENCES

1. Robot Timeline—Robotic History. RobotWorx. Available at: http://www.used-robots.com/robot-education.php?page=robot+timeline. Accessed May 31, 2011.
2. Robot History: Isaac Asimov. RobotWorx. Available at: http://www.used-robots.com/robot-education.php?page=asimov. Accessed May 31, 2011.
3. HeartLander. Carnegie Mellon Robotics Institute. Available at: http://www.ri.cmu.edu/research_project_detail.html?project_id=533&menu_id=261. Accessed May 31, 2011.

Preface

Robotic Surgery is Here to Stay

When I was in nursing school going through the many rotations of Medicine, Pediatrics, Orthopedics, Geriatrics, and others, I always wondered where I was going to end up. One day my nursing instructor came to me and said, "Tomorrow will be your day in surgery, you will follow a nurse in the OR". I showed up the next day and watched. I knew then what my nursing career would be. When I started my first job in the OR, I was amazed and excited to be there; it was just as I imagined, large open cases with good visibility of anatomy.

When my family moved and I had to take another job at a much smaller hospital, I was surprised at how technologically advanced they were. The first case I witnessed was a laparoscopic bowel resection. I had never seen a laparoscopic bowel resection in the large city hospital, only open resections. During my introduction to advancing technology in surgery, robotic surgery was emerging as the new player on the forefront. It started in urology with prostate surgery. The advancements kept coming in the fields of gynecology, cardiac, and general surgery. All these areas have played a role in the advancement of robotic surgery. In today's OR it may be hard not to find a surgical robot in a large metropolitan surgery department. We are even finding surgical robots in midsize and rural hospitals.

A wide range of topics is covered in this issue on robotic surgery: Dr David Chou and Dr Phillip Mucksavage introduce a topic familiar with Robotic Surgery—Laparscopic-Assisted Robotic Prostatectomy. Dr Chou and Dr Mucksavage review the process of patient selection and intraoperative details of a Robotic Prostatectomy, as well as costs, patient satisfaction, and outcomes. They also discuss a newer area in robotic surgery—Robotic-Assisted Renal Surgery, covering techniques and potential issues associated with Robotic Renal Surgery.

We also look at the process a rural hospital took in developing a successful robotic surgery program. With large city markets saturated with hospitals being able to perform robotic surgeries, we tend to forget the large rural population having to drive long distances to a major city to receive robotic surgery and follow-up care. This rural hospital decided it was time to bring quality robotic surgical care to its coverage area.

Robotic surgery, like all other types of surgeries, is constantly evolving. New models join old models; old models get upgrades, software, and instrumentation changes. How does a surgery department keep up with these changes and properly train its staff? Rena Thompson, RN, MSN, CNS-BC, and Mariana Boyle, RN, BSN, CNOR, discuss how they used electronic learning to cover training, tackle issues, and track staff competencies.

Two additional articles cover nursings' most important issue: the Patient! Cynthia Thomas, RN, BSN, CNOR, discusses the importance of patient positioning. During Robotic Surgery, the patient can be put in some awkward positions. Making sure the patient is protected and safe is the highest priority we have as circulators.

Perioperative Nursing Clinics 6 (2011) xi–xii
doi:10.1016/j.cpen.2011.06.008

Christina Thell, RN, BSN, CNOR, studies pre- and postprocedure perceptions patients and families have regarding robotic surgery and how the perioperative nurse can play a significant role in easing patient and family anxieties for a patient going through a robotic surgical procedure.

Robotic surgery is here to stay. As technology advances, robotic surgery will be sure to follow with new procedures and techniques. Staying up to date on robotic surgery and its advancements and keeping the patient first in our priorities will help us all stay ahead of the game.

John Zender, RN, BS, CNOR
St Joseph's Medical Center
523 North Third Street
Brainerd, MN 56401, USA

E-mail address:
jzenderorrn@yahoo.com

Keeping Pace with Robotic Technology

Rena Thompson, RN, MSN, CNS-BC, Mariana Boyle, RN, BSN, CNOR

KEYWORDS

• Robotic • Education • Training

Surgical robots were introduced to the industry in 1985. The idea of telesurgery was principally developed by the military, with the intention of allowing surgeons to treat wounded soldiers miles away.[1] Robots entered the surgery arena in the field of urology in the 1980s for transurethral resection of the prostate. Unfortunately, because of poor ultrasound imaging of the prostate, it was not a preferred treatment. Also, in 1985, robots were used for intraoperative percutaneous renal procedures.[2] The first robot approved by the Food and Drug Administration was the ROBODOC (Curexo Technology Corporation, Fremont, CA, USA). Since then, robots have been used in different procedures in surgery—from neurosurgical biopsies to hip replacements.[3]

There have been different types of robotic systems over the years: the Puma 560 (Unimation), PROBOT (Imperial College, London), and ROBODOC. Each robot was able to provide a greater precision for the surgeon in the surgical procedure.[3] In the late 1990s and early 2000s, 2 different robotic systems appeared in the surgical arena: da Vinci (Intuitive Surgical; Sunnyvale, CA, USA) and Zeus (Computer Motion; Santa Barbara, CA, USA).[4] These are the 2 robotic systems approved in the United States for laparoscopic thoracoscopic surgery.[2] In many of the surgical adult and pediatric procedures, the robotic surgical system has been approved for use.[2] Along with the development of robotic surgery, the practice and associated training of intraoperative nurses evolved as well.

At the University of Chicago Medical Center (UCMC), we are performing robotic procedures in the following services: adult and pediatric urology, gynecology, cardiac, thoracic, and general surgery. In the near future, robotic surgeries will be expanding to vascular surgery.

ROBOTIC TECHNOLOGY CHANGES

Currently, Intuitive owns the Zeus and da Vinci robots.[4] In 2000, Intuitive received approval for their standard robotic system. The standard system included a vision cart, patient cart, and ergonomic surgeon console. Intuitive updated their systems (S, Si) to include a motorized patient cart, high-speed fiber optic connections, improved

University of Chicago Medical Center, 5841 South Maryland Avenue, MC # 1083, Chicago, IL 60645, USA

E-mail address: Rena.Thompson@uchospitals.edu

Perioperative Nursing Clinics 6 (2011) 201–212
doi:10.1016/j.cpen.2011.05.002
1556-7931/11/$ – see front matter © 2011 Elsevier Inc. All rights reserved.

arm range of motion, integrated touchscreen, and multiple other upgrades. The upgrades provided the surgeon and surgical team with the ability to maneuver the robot, allowing precise surgery (**Table 1**). With the changes in robotic system technologies, draping the da Vinci became straightforward. Attached components were added to the drapes, ie, camera and instrument arm. This streamlined the robot setup time for the surgical team (**Table 2**).

INTRAOPERATIVE ROBOTIC NURSING EDUCATION HISTORY

With the evolution of robotic technology, a need was identified to provide intraoperative staff with initial and continued robotic training. Some of the initial methods of education were on-the-job training. For example, in the early 2000s at UCMC, the manufacturer provided an inservice presented by a manufacturer technician. The inservice included an overview of the system, draping, and cable connections. The manufacturer also provided off-site training, which became problematic because of institutional restraints including staff scheduling, time, and personnel. The off-site training was not consistent with the overall nursing needs[11] and focused on the needs of the surgical case but not the overall robotic system.

There is a need for providing the staff with consistent information, and formalized in-house training provides a process for ensuring competency for assisting robotic surgery.

NURSING EDUCATION BACKGROUND

Continuing nursing education has historically been based on acquiring new knowledge and using various methods (lectures, hands-on, and so forth) to instruct the nurse in new skills and updated knowledge base. Every nurse has a different way of achieving competency and assessment of skills. An experienced nurse's skills will be much different than a nurse with limited skills.

Traditionally, education has included different formats, for example, traditional lectures, observation and demonstration, interactive teaching, and facilitator roles.[12] Group education creates a beneficial environment for the nurses to review new knowledge and exchange information.[13] The use of interdisciplinary training provides collaboration of knowledge for the staff nurses and extends their experiences beyond their current educational horizons.[13]

The nursing education community has seen an increase of electronic learning. A format of electronic learning is the use of computer-based modules (online modules) to enhance and assist the nurse's knowledge base. In 2000, approximately 80% of training in the workplace was completed via classroom. Over the last 10 years this number has dropped and has been replaced with electronic learning.[14]

In 1982, Benner published "Novice to Expert Theory." In her theory, she emphasizes that a nurse develops skills and knowledge over a time continuum within the aspects of experiences. The levels of nursing experience that she listed are novice, advanced beginner, competent, proficient, and expert.[15] Benner defines each level as the following:

- Novice: no experience in the task or skill[16]
- Advance beginner: has enough hands-on experience to perform the skill but may not be able to see the larger perspective[16]
- Competent: usually has a couple years of experience and is able to plan deliberately for the hands-on experience[16]
- Proficient: usually has the ability to perceive the situation and skill as a whole and is able to use past experience to troubleshoot and modify plans as needed[16]
- Expert: does not rely on the abstract and skills knowledge. The expert knows the skill intuitively and is able to plan fluidly as need arises.[16]

Table 1
Types of da Vinci robots

Standard	S	Si
3 Robotic arms	4 Robotic arms	4 Robotic arms
1 Camera	1 Camera	1 Camera
Components • Surgeon console • Vision cart • Surgical cart	Components • Surgeon console • Vision cart • Patient cart	Components • Surgeon console • Vision cart • Patient cart
Surgical cart • Nonmotorized • Not identified as the "patient cart"[5] • Need 2 staff to move[5]	Patient cart • Name change from surgical cart to patient cart • Motor drive • Sweet spot blue bar identified • Need 2 staff to move • Operates manually[6]	Patient cart • Throttle, plus • Same as S[7]
Attaching cables: Cable connections: Cables: • Surgical cart to Surgeon console × 3 • Vision cart cables × 4 to surgeon console[5]	Attaching cables: Cable connections: Cables: • Surgical cart to Surgeon console × 1 • Vision cart cables × 2 to surgeon console[6]	Attaching cables: Cable connections: • Cables to connect vision cart to patient cart/surgeon console are interchangeable[7]
Surgeon console 2D[5]	Surgeon console 2D and 3D, HD[6]	Surgeon console 3D, HD[7]
Powering up Press green system button[5]	Powering up Via green power button • Integrated mode: Power on surgical console will power up patient cart. • Stand-alone mode: Individual power up of patient cart and surgeon's console[6]	Powering up Stand-alone mode (see S)[7]
Calibration endoscope • only via surgeon console[8]	Calibration endoscope • options: surgeon console or touchscreen[6]	Calibration endoscope • can initiate via 3D camera head and vision cart touch screen[7]

(continued on next page)

Table 1
(continued)

Standard	S	Si
Calibration of camera • white balance via the vision cart, camera control units[5]	**Calibration of camera** • same as Standard[6]	**Calibration of camera** • via camera head or vision cart touch screen[7]
Homing • initiated via surgeon console, powered by ready button; • ensure surgical cart & surgeon console arms are separated; • 3 beeps = self-test completion and ready[5]	**Homing** • Must remove arms from stow position; initiated via surgeon console, press HOME button located on surgeon console. • 3 beeps = self-test completion and ready[6]	**Homing** • Must remove arms from stow position; once all components (vision cart, patient cart, and surgeon's console) are fully powered up, homing is automatic[7]
Instrument arm LEDs Icons: displayed on assistant monitor and surgeon console display (ie, bright blue: ready for surgeon console control; white side-to-side blinking: clutching, etc)[5]	**Instrument arm LEDs** Each instrument arm has LED lights that indicate a fault/ready for use (ie, bright blue: ready for surgeon console control; side-to-side blinking white: clutching; etc)[6]	**Instrument arm LEDs** Same as S[7]
EndoWrist Instrument Tracking: end of case system displays summary table of remaining lives of EndoWrist instruments and EndoWrist sterile adapter[5]	**EndoWrist Instrument** Tracking: Monitor will display # of EndoWrist instrument lives remaining when instrument is engaged and summary table at end of case[6]	**EndoWrist Instrument** Tracking: use touchscreen to find utilities tab/ press inventory management button to view the remaining EndoWrist instrument lives at any time during the case[7]
System shut down • Fold surgical (instrument and camera) arms against surgical cart • Press the system button on surgeon console • Power off vision cart and unplug cables from surgeon console and store on vision cart • Unplug cables on surgeon console and store on surgical cart • Surgeon console must be plugged in while stored[5]	**System shut down** • Stow third instrument arm • Fold the instrument and camera arms against the patient cart • Press power button on surgeon console • Power off illuminator and the vision cart (locate switch on the isolation transformer) • Disconnect cables (cables are stored on the vision cart and patient cart[6]	**System shut down** • Stow third instrument arm • Fold the instrument and camera arms against the patient cart • Press any system power button • Disconnect system cables and store with protective caps[9]

Table 2
Draping changes

	Standard	S	Si
Instrument arm	Insert and attach sterile adaptor manually[8]	Pre-attached adaptor to sterile drape[6]	Pre-attached adaptor to sterile drape[7]
Cannula mount instrument	Manually attached to instrument arm[5]	Pre-attached to instrument arm[6]	Pre-attached to instrument arm[7]
Camera	• Pre-attached camera sterile adaptor to endoscope before draping • drape endoscope[8]	Same as standard[10]	Sterile adapter camera arm is integrated with drape[7]
Camera arm	Sterile adapter camera arm attached to camera arm drape adhesive, then firmly attached to endoscope[8]	Same as standard[10]	Sterile adapter camera arm is integrated with drape[7]
Cannula mount camera	Attached to the camera arm (the drape molds to it).[6]	Manually attached to camera arm[8]	Same as S[7]

The levels of nursing experiences are fluid and may change depending on the skill and situation. A nurse may be an expert in one area, but when placed in an unfamiliar skill set or case may revert back to the novice level until further training or experience move her back through the levels to competent or expert.[16]

TRAINING

In 2009, UCMC owned the 3 types of da Vinci robots. All are different robotic generations (Standard, S, and Si). After the purchase of the Si, the intraoperative clinical education department realized there was a knowledge deficit among the robotic nurses who were trained on the Standard da Vinci robot. Clinical nursing education identified the necessity of an informal needs assessment with the introduction of the new generation da Vinci robotic system. When UCMC upgraded and purchased the Si system, the robotic-trained staff members' nursing skill levels reverted back to the novice nursing skill level. The UCMC robotic training was designed to assist the nurses in progressing from novice to competent nurses in the robotic Si system.

UCMC has used online education as a primary or secondary educational tool. Computer-based modules (online modules) create an increased environment of learning for the healthcare institution. Because of the scheduling of cases in an operating room setting, the intraoperative nurses have limited time to complete classroom training. The online modules have provided another avenue to provide training and information to the nurses within a reasonable timeframe.[17]

Other advantages to online modules include:

- Training cost reduction because of increased staff access to the online learning activity[18]
- Self-paced learning[19]
- Convenient time and location[17]
- Introduction to initial knowledge-based concepts[17]
- Instructor's ability to expand and reinforce online module concepts versus initial knowledge.[17]

Disadvantages of using the online modules include:

- Knowledge of basic computer skills[20]
- Internet connectivity[20]
- Computer availability and access[20]
- Hardware and software problems[20]
- Need of continual initial and ongoing technical support[20]
- Learner may not independently complete online module[17]
- Instructors unfamiliar with online module content[17]
- Learner unable to retain the content of the online module.[17]

The UCMC has provided online module access to the staff nurses and surgical technicians because of the advantages stated above. The online modules provided a foundation and reinforcement of knowledge for the operating room nurses, so their hands-on skills lab would be beneficial to them.

The online modules were a requirement for the staff members to complete within a predetermined timeline of 30 days. The online modules provided staff members a knowledge foundation to prepare them for the interactive/hands-on robotic training.[17]

The online modules included the following topics:

1. System overview (ie, reviews the surgeon's console, patient cart, and vision cart)
2. Operating room set up and system connections (cable connections and system power up)
3. Draping (ie, camera and instrument arm[s])
4. Docking (ie, finding the sweet spot)
5. Vision cart overview (ie, components, touchscreen monitor, camera control unit [CCU], etc.)
6. Safety features (ie, system faults, troubleshooting, emergency stop, error logs, etc.).

Another education mode of delivery is to blend online training with the traditional interactive/classroom training.[17] During robotic training, UCMC used the electronic learning in the format of online modules to assist in the didactic training of the participants.

Advantages of blended classroom and online training include the following:

- Interactive classroom[17]
- Additional time and flexibility to increase the interactive content in the classroom.[17]

It was determined that training should include observation and demonstration with didactic built in to reinforce foundational concepts of the online modules and robotic system. The initial course was with the multidisciplinary team of experts invited from the robotic company to provide the needed hands-on and didactic training for the staff. During the subsequent classes, proficient/expert (super users) robotic-trained staff member(s) provided hands-on and didactic training to staff members.

During the classroom hands-on sessions, staff members had the opportunity to practice and demonstrate the basic robotic functionalities. At the end of the classroom period, competency validation checklists were used to document staff's performance (**Fig. 1**). The competency validation checklists is an outline for the training class. Each participant reviews and demonstrates each performance validation technique. The competency validation checklist includes the ability to identify the major components of the da Vinci system, instruments, power up, cable connections, draping, and so forth.

UCMC disadvantages of classroom training include the following:

- Limited number of participants
- Scheduled time and location of training
- Instructor time and cost.

Staff members were assigned to a preceptor for the hands-on experiences using the competency validation checklist for a guide to their hands-on training (see **Fig. 1**).

ROBOTIC TRAINING ISSUES

The robotic training provides opportunities of daily improvement in skill levels. The hands-on training included many common issues and troubleshooting. The following areas were identified during training as potential issues or errors that are common to the novice skill level:

- Connection of cables to vision cart–patient cart–surgeon console (ie, S systems are not interchangeable)[6,7]

UNIVERSITY OF CHICAGO MEDICAL CENTER
DEPARTMENT OF NURSING
OPERATING ROOM EQUIPMENT CHECKLIST

	da Vinci Robot Competency VALIDATION Checklist Part II
	GOAL: Demonstrates competency in managing DaVinci S System intraoperatively
	1. Identifies LED Status Indicator Lights
	A. Able t o identify when surgeon is ready to control DaVinci System by using LED status indicators.
	B. Able t o identify when an intervention to the DaVinci S System is required using LED Status Indicator Lights.
	1) Yellow light – intervention is required
	2) Red light – system restart is required
	3) Fast blinking green light – downloads for new instrument information are available
	4) Bright blue light – ready for surgeon control
	5) Alternate side to side blinking green – guided tool change
	6) Solid white – not ready for surgeon
	7) Alternate side to side blinking white - clutching

References:
Intuitive Surgical. da Vinci Surgical System User Manual. Sunnyvale, CA: Intuitive Surgical; 2007
da vinci S system overview script **www.davincisurgerycommunity.com** April 8, 2011.

Name (print): _____   Date: _____

Signature (if applicable): _____

Fig. 1. Robot competency validation checklist.

- Camera head connection to the endoscope and calibration (ie, white balance: S system on the CCU vs Si on the CCU and camera head)[6,7]
- Endoscope calibration with alignment tool (ie, endoscope needs to calibrate up and down with the use of calibration alignment tool)[6,7]
- Clutching and movement of the patient cart's instrument and camera arms (ie, operator unfamiliar with different clutching and movement control of the camera and instrument arm joints)[6,7]
- Draping of instrument and camera arms without contamination (ie, potential contamination when placing the drape on the camera and instrument arms)[6,7]
- Troubleshooting EndoWrist (Intuitive Surgical; Sunnyvale, CA, USA) instrument issues: inadvertent tightening of tip on tissue (use emergency wrench); tracking remaining lives; and proper storage of tips (ie, S system displays the EndoWrist instrument's lives when engaged, or summarizes at end of case vs Si operator may review lives anytime during case)[6,7]

Name _____ Service _____ Procedures: _____   1

OR SCRUB EXPERIENCE GOALS

DATE	GOALS	PERFORMANCE	ACTION
	To be able to scrub independently on surgical procedures.	Document goal met or goal not met	If goal not meet, the manager/educator documents what the next steps are.
	1. Can set-up the sterile field independently.		
	2. Knows the names of all instruments on each case.		
	3. Performs draping procedure.		
	4. Knows sequencing of procedure.		
	5. Anticipates surgeons needs.		
	6. Hands suture smoothly and receives back safely.		
	7. Demonstrates proper handling of the following staples, ie hemoclips, if applicable		
	8. Initiates & performs correct sponge and needle counts.		
	9. Passes instruments safely & according to surgeon preference.		
	10. Appropriately reassembles trays in preparation for decontamination process (ie removes bioburden)		
	11. Appropriately handles specimens		
	12. Follows Medication Safety NPSG: • labels all medications • labels one med. at a time • labeling includes name, strength, amount • verifies meds. with circ. nurse		

Employee Signatures _____

To be completed by preceptor

To be completed by manager/educator

_____ Evaluator Signature

Fig. 2. Assessment checklist.

- Docking: finding the sweet spot to line up the patient cart to the correct patient position (ie, unable to line up the sweet spot to the sterile field and patient position).[6,7]

TRACKING STAFF EXPERIENCES

Staff members are assigned to a preceptor for hands-on experiences. Each surgical experience is documented on a daily scrub goal form (**Fig. 2**). The scrub goal form provides procedural goals for the staff member in training. At the end of the procedure, the preceptor reviews and documents whether the goals are met. Once all the goals are met for a procedural experience, the date is documented on the robotic rotational checklist (**Fig. 3**). The preceptor's signature indicates that the staff member has demonstrated the ability to scrub and/or circulate independently. This determination was in collaboration with the preceptor, manager, and educator/designee. The timeframe was dependent on case volume and individual learning styles.

IDEAL CONTINUED NURSING EDUCATION

The ideal classroom robot education for nursing includes simulation. This format provides hands-on practice sessions, without the risk of patient injury. Simulation also provides opportunities for the different nursing skill levels, from novice to expert, to practice in a realistic robotic surgical case. It provides an opportunity for the interdisciplinary surgical team to practice common and uncommon clinical robotic system experiences such as troubleshooting robotic faults, converting to open procedures, inadvertent system shutdown, and so forth.

University of Chicago Medical Center
Rotational Checklists
Robot

S=scrub
C=circulate

Name: _____

Please Log all procedures completed by date. Also indicate scrub or circulate.

Preceptor(s):					
Procedures:	Date	Date	Date	N/A	Signature
GU: Nephrectomy					
GU: Prostatectomy					
GU: other					
GU Peds: ureteral implant					
GU peds:other					
GYNE: Assisted Hysterectomy					
Thoracic					
GEN: parathyroids					
General- Colectomy					
Vascular					
Cardiac					

Preceptor signature indicates that the staff member demonstrated ability to scrub and circulate independently.

Equipment	Date	Date	Date	N/A	Signature
electrocautery					
robot: console					
robot: video tower					
robot: patient cart					
robot instrumentation					
robot endowrists					
robot instrumentation: precleaning					

Preceptor signature indicates that the staff member demonstrated ability to scrub and circulate independently.

Fig. 3. Rotational checklist.

Simulation is becoming the wave of the future for the education of nurses and interdisciplinary team training. It is the instruction of clinical knowledge, skills, and clinical elements that can be transferred to the actual clinical setting.[21] In the past, nurses have learned clinical skills at the bedside, which increased the risk of errors on clinical patients.[22] The use of simulation provides the ability for the learner to make mistakes without the risk of harming the patient. It can provide benefits in interdisciplinary healthcare team training by providing an accurate clinical situation and evaluation of communication, assessment, diagnosis, and treatment of a clinical patient.[23]

Simulation provides an environment for the nurse and healthcare team to clinical conditions and situations that may not be addressed during clinical training.[22] The two different types of simulation are low and high fidelity. Fidelity refers to the accuracy or reality of the reproduction from the original source. Therefore, high fidelity is more accurate than low.[21] Low-fidelity simulation refers to the instruction of psychomotor skills. High fidelity, on the other hand, refers to the instruction of complex education objectives, ie, resuscitation, airway emergencies, and operating room team training.[24] Simulation has three primary teaching modes: scenario, simulator, and the experience. The scenario should be scripted out to provide the participants with a realistic clinical situation. The simulator should imitate the patient responses, physical space, and equipment to the actual clinical event and setting. The experience should provide the participants the reality of the clinical setting.[23] Simulation should also include a debriefing time for the nurses to review their responses during the clinical event. At times, video recording is another way to provide accurate feedback to the nurses or healthcare team.[22,25]

Once initial training has been validated for the staff member or surgical team, annual robotic education should be assessed. If possible, conduct annual competency validation of hands-on skill to ensure the staff is up to date with their robotic skills.[11] The UCMC future plan is that robotic-trained staff members should undertake an annual completion of online modules, validation of hands-on skills, and any robotic system changes and revisions. Robotic-trained staff should have ongoing support through actual robot assignments with the support of a preceptor. The team should also be prepared for the plan of action if a procedure converts to an open procedure, ie, emergency open prostatectomy.

SUMMARY

UCMC has successfully trained staff members on the S and Si robot systems using the interactive blended training format. The success in training was due to the online, hands-on interactive blended training, and preceptor participation. The future continued robotic education plan includes incorporating interdisciplinary simulation with the interactive blended modalities. This will provide opportunities for all to maintain the pace of robotic technology.

REFERENCES

1. Guidarelli M. Robotic surgery. The next generation: an introduction to medicine 2006;2(4). Available at: http://www.nextgenmd.org/vol2-5/robotic_surgery. Accessed November 4, 2010.
2. Francis P, Winfield H. Medical robotics: the impact on perioperative nursing practice. Urol Nurs 2006;26(2):99–108.
3. Lanfranco A, Castellanos A, Desai J, et al. Robotic surgery: a current perspective. Ann Surg 2004;239(1):14–21.
4. Zender J, Thell C. Developing a successful robotic surgery program. AORN J 2010;92(1):72–86.
5. da Vinci standard system overview script. Available at: http://www.davincisurgerycommunity.com. Accessed April 6, 2011.
6. da Vinci S system overview script. Available at: http://www.davincisurgerycommunity.com. Accessed April 8, 2011.
7. da Vinci Si system overview script. Available at: http://www.davincisurgerycommunity.com. Accessed March 30, 2011.
8. Intuitive Surgical. The da Vinci endoscopic instrument control system user manual. Sunnyvale, California: Intuitive Surgical, Inc; 2001. p. 3–7.
9. Intuitive Surgical. da Vinci surgical system user manual. Sunnyvale (CA): Intuitive Surgical; 2007. p. 4–10.
10. Intuitive Surgical. da Vinci surgical system Si user manual. Sunnyvale (CA): Intuitive Surgical; 2009. p. 11–4.

11. Francis P. The evolution of robotics in surgery and implementing a perioperative robotics nurse specialist role. AORN J 2006;83(3):629–50.
12. Marzlin K. Structuring continuing education to change practice a nurse driven initiative. Dimens Crit Care Nurs 2011;30(1):41–52.
13. Purcell S. Transformational learning in the perioperative setting. Pfiedler Enterprises 2010;8222:9–17.
14. Ratka J. Journey to Oz: the yellow brick road to a blended learning environment. Crit Care Nurs Quart 2010;33(1):35–43.
15. Benner PE. From novice to expert. Nurs Theories 2010. Available at: http://currentnursing.com/nursing_theory/Patricia_Benner_From_Novice_to_Expert.html. Accessed March 17, 2011.
16. Mitre J, Alexander J. Keller S. Patricia Benner: From novice to expert: excellence and power in clinical nursing practice. In: Alligood MR, Tomey AM, editors. Nursing theorists and their work. 4th edition. St. Louis: Mosby, Elsevier; 1998. p. 157–72.
17. Bradley C, Erice M, Halfer D, et al. The impact of a blended learning approach on instructor and learner satisfaction with preceptor education. J Nurses Staff Dev 2007;23(4):164–70.
18. Walsh K, Rafiq I, Hall R. Online education tools developed by heart improve the knowledge and skills of hospital doctors in cardiology. Postgrad Med J 2007;83: 502–3.
19. Kozlowski D. Using online learning in a traditional face to face environment. Comput Nurs 2002;20(1):23–30.
20. Lu D, Lin Z, Li Y. Effects of a web-based course on nursing skills and knowledge learning. J Nurs Educ 2009;48(2):70–7.
21. Andreatta P, Bullough A, Marzano D. Simulation and team training. Clin Obst Gynecol 2010;53(3):532–44.
22. Fort C, Fitzgerald B. How simulation improves perioperative nursing. OR Nurs 2011;March:36–42.
23. Cates L. Simulation training: a multidisciplinary approach. Adv Neonatal Care 2011; 11(2):95–100.
24. Turban J. Peters D, Berg B. Live defibrillation in simulation-based medical education—a survey of simulation center practices and attitudes. Simulation in Healthcare 2010;5(1):24–7.
25. Corriveau C. Learner-centered simulated training: just what the patient ordered. Crit Care Med 2010;38(9):1916–8.

Developing a Successful Robotic Surgery Program in a Rural Hospital

John Zender, RN, BS, CNOR*, Christina G. Thell, RN, BSN, CNOR

KEYWORDS

- Robotic surgery program • Rural health care facilities
- Laparoscopic surgery • Robotic advantages

The development of robotic surgery has been one of the greatest advances in surgical technology since the introduction of minimally invasive surgery via laparoscopes. Robotic surgery was introduced in 1985 with the PUMA 560, which was used to orient a needle for a brain biopsy under computed tomography guidance.[1] Today, the robotic surgical system has become a common tool for laparoscopic surgeries in major metropolitan hospitals, and with a rapidly expanding market, rural health care facilities now have the opportunity to offer their patients the latest technology in laparoscopic surgery as well.

Although the initial financial obligation is large, a robotics program can give a hospital a competitive advantage in becoming a leader in exceptional care. Purchasing the technology alone is not enough. Developing a robotics program requires intense training, marketing, and the dedication and passion of surgical team members ready to take their surgical care to the next level. With a well-developed robotics program, a hospital has the opportunity for great financial success in addition to providing patients with cutting-edge health care. This article details the implementation of a robotics program at St Joseph's Medical Center in the rural community of Brainerd, Minnesota.

Evolution of Surgical Robots

Three influential groups of professionals initially developed the concept of using robotic technology in surgery during the late 1980s. First, scientists at the National Aeronautics and Space Administration (NASA), in Washington, DC, incorporated telepresence into medicine by developing virtual reality.[1,2] This enabled surgeons to be completely enveloped in their surgical field through the use of a computer. When the surgeon looks through the surgeon console, he or she sees only what the

This article was previously published in the July 2010 issue of *AORN journal*.
Disclosure: The authors have nothing to disclose.
St Joseph's Medical Center, 523 North Third Street, Brainerd, MN 56401, USA
* Corresponding author.
E-mail address: jzenderorrn@yahoo.com

Perioperative Nursing Clinics 6 (2011) 213–225
doi:10.1016/j.cpen.2011.06.007

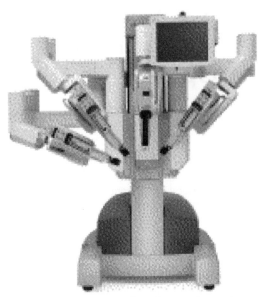

Fig. 1. The da Vinci surgical robot also is referred to as the patient cart. Instruments are attached to the working arms and advanced through trocars to the surgical site. (Photograph *courtesy of* Intuitive Surgical, Inc, Sunnyvale, CA.)

endoscope is aimed at and does not have the background distractions that can occur during a typical surgical procedure.

Next, a group of scientists from Stanford Research Institute, Menlo Park, California, teamed with NASA to establish telemanipulation.[1,3,4] This technology can replicate human hand motions through movement of the robotic instrument arms. This caught the attention of a general surgery endoscopist who was working for the US Army.[1] The endoscopist saw the benefits of using robotic technology to perform surgery on soldiers in combat zones. The US Army provided funding for medical robotics and was instrumental in the development of the technology.[1]

The first independent company to gain US Food and Drug Administration (FDA) approval to market and sell a medical robotic system was Computer Motion, Inc.[1] In 1994, Computer Motion launched AESOP (Automated Endoscopic System for Optimal Positioning), a robotic telescope manipulator.[1] In 1995, a second company, Intuitive Surgical, Inc, joined the market.[1,4] Intuitive Surgical developed and began marketing the da Vinci Robotic Surgical System in 2000 (**Fig. 1**).[4] In 2001, Computer Motion began marketing ZEUS, a complete robotic system.[1] Intuitive Surgical purchased Computer Motion in 2003 and now owns rights to the only 2 FDA-approved robotic surgical systems in the United States: da Vinci and ZEUS.[1,4] "Today there are more than 1,482 da Vinci Systems installed in 1,151 hospitals worldwide" (A. Morgan, MarCom Manager, Intuitive Surgical, Inc; e-mail communication; April 18, 2010).

Description of the Robotic System

The surgical robot is a "collection of wristed servant tools called manipulators, which receive digital instructions from an interfaced computer . . . The manipulators inside the patient's body duplicate the surgeon's hand movements at the

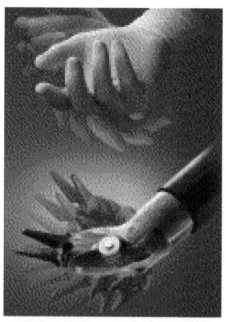

Fig. 2. The manipulators duplicate the surgeon's hand motions at the surgeon console. (Photograph *courtesy of* Intuitive Surgical, Inc, Sunnyvale, CA.)

console"[2] (**Fig. 2**). The system consists of 3 main pieces: the surgeon console, the patient cart, and the vision cart (**Fig. 3**). After the surgeon places the trocars in the desired anatomic location and achieves optimal visualization, guided docking of the robotic arms occurs as the patient cart is moved into position over the patient.

A   **B**   **C**

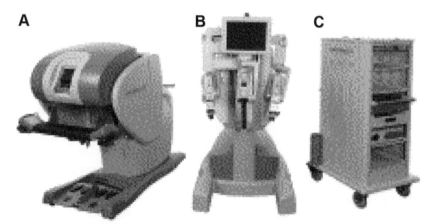

Fig. 3. The da Vinci surgical system. From left to right are the surgeon console where the surgeon sits to perform the procedure (*A*); the patient cart, which holds the instrumentation (*B*); and the vision cart, which houses the camera, light source, and other ancillary equipment such as the electrosurgical unit (*C*). (Photograph *courtesy of* Intuitive Surgical, Inc, Sunnyvale, CA.)

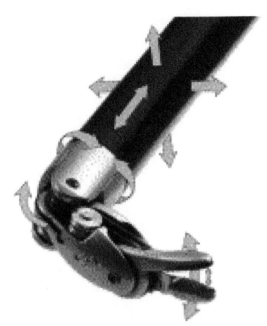

Fig. 4. The robotic instruments are wristed (ie, jointed) in seven degrees of freedom. (Photograph *courtesy of* Intuitive Surgical, Inc, Sunnyvale, CA.)

Typically, guided docking is performed by the circulating nurse, who moves the robotic arms over the patient. The surgeon then guides them to the precise location so the robotic instruments line up parallel to the trocars. The surgeon attaches the instrument and camera arms to the trocars and places the instrument into the cavity. The surgeon leaves the sterile field and sits at the surgeon console, where he or she performs the procedure. Currently, the FDA mandates that all surgical robots must be controlled by a surgeon who is in the same room as the patient.[5]

Just as laparoscopy has dramatically changed patient outcomes, so does robotic surgery. In addition to providing all the benefits of laparoscopic procedures such as shorter hospital stays, decreased pain, and fewer postoperative complications, using a surgical robot can overcome the disadvantages of traditional laparoscopic surgery. The surgical robot offers the surgeon a 3-dimensional view, ergonomic advantages, increased dexterity, and the ability to perform microsurgery.[5]

The surgeon has a 3-dimensional view of the surgical field through 2 cameras, or "eyes," in the same scope. This increases the surgeon's visual and depth perception and mimics the traditional open surgical approach. The surgeon is able to sit comfortably at the console for the majority of the procedure with padded armrests and a height-specific field of vision. This decreases fatigue, reduces loss of instrument control, and increases the surgeon's ability to fully concentrate on the procedure at hand.

The robot mimics and improves movements of the human wrist, hands, and fingers. The technology has the ability to filter out the natural hand tremors that a surgeon can experience, which can become magnified in traditional laparoscopic surgery. The robotic instruments are wristed (ie, jointed) in 7 degrees of freedom (**Fig. 4**). This greatly aids in fine dissection and delicate suturing. The robotic system increases magnification, which allows earlier detection of bleeding, and increases dexterity, which allows for precise vein ligation. This in turn results in less overall blood loss for the patient and decreases the risk of the need for transfusion.

By using the robot in laparoscopic procedures, surgery can be performed on considerably smaller regions of the body than in conventional procedures. For instance, although the prostate is located deep in the pelvis, it is easily accessed with robotic instrumentation.

One question is often asked: Does the surgeon have tactile sensation, known as *haptics*, while performing robotic surgery? The answer is yes and no. "The robotic surgical system relays some force feedback sensations from the surgical field back to the surgeon throughout the procedure. This force feedback provides a substitute for tactile sensation. This feedback is augmented by the enhanced vision provided by the high-resolution 3D-view."[6(p3)] According to Intuitive Surgical, after the surgeon performs a number of robotic procedures and becomes comfortable with the surgeon console and robotic functions, a "visual haptics" occurs. This means that the surgeon achieves a level of comfort with the visual stimulation provided by the ability to view in 3 dimensions, high definition, and increased magnification, which can compensate for the loss of tactile stimulation.[7]

Market Research

The first step in setting up a robotic surgery program at any facility, but particularly in a rural area, is to perform market research of the geographic area. This helps determine whether there is a potential need for robotic surgeries and whether the program will be successful in a particular setting. In most cases, a state's hospital association can provide market share information on the types of procedures being performed in the coverage area of a facility. For rural hospitals, this area typically ranges from a 50- to 100-mile radius. From that information, health care facility administrators can determine the number of surgical patients that have come from the coverage area and whether the facility has lost any of these patients to a competing hospital or facility in a larger city.

At St Joseph's Medical Center, the nearest robotic surgical hospital is 70 miles south and 2 others are 150 miles away, 1 to the northwest and 1 to the northeast. When we conducted market research, we discovered that we were losing a percentage of the market share to facilities with robotics programs. We determined that a robotics program would benefit our hospital to gain back that market share, increase productivity, and provide a needed service to our area communities.

If the market research indicates that a program is needed, the next important step is to find out whether surgical staff members are interested in performing robotic procedures. One urologist who performed surgery at our facility had robotic training. For a rural hospital to rely solely on one surgical field of practice to support a robotic surgery program would result in failure of the program because not enough procedures could be performed to pay for the investment in the robot and required staff training. Fortunately, we had another urologist, 3 obstetrician/gynecologists, and 2 general surgeons willing to be trained in robotic surgery. With 3 surgical services on board, we determined that launching a robotics program in our rural facility would be possible.

It may be wise to ask the surgeons who undergo robotics training to sign an agreement (ie, a noncompete clause) that after they are trained, they will commit to the organization and only perform robotic surgery in that health care organization. This may not be a problem in a rural community where surgeons may only practice at 1 or 2 health care facilities.

Financing

For a small hospital, obtaining financing for a $2 million robot is not an easy task and can make or break a robotic surgery program. Nevertheless, many different ways to obtain financing are available to rural hospitals; finding one that meets the needs of the institution can be key in acquiring a surgical robot. Examples of funding sources include the following:

- State and federal programs
- Foundation grants
- Donations
- Government programs (ie, economic stimulus package)
- Grateful patient programs or memorials
- Employees and physician donations (eg, monthly paycheck deductions)
- Loans.

In our case, the chief executive officer appealed to the St Joseph's Foundation for funding because its board members live in the community and use the services of the hospital. The reasons that we cited for adding a robotic surgery program included

- A noted decrease in surgeries because some that were regularly performed at our facility were being lost to other hospitals where the same surgeries were being performed robotically
- The ability to draw and retain talented surgeons by having robotic surgery available in our facility
- The growing trend of robotic surgery expanding to rural areas, making it more likely that if we did not obtain a surgical robot, one of our competitors might.

St Joseph's Foundation granted us the money to purchase the robot. To thank the Foundation for its donation, we provided recognition in our monthly facility newsletter, in advertising, and at board meetings.

Program Development

To implement a new program at any facility, a multidisciplinary steering committee should be assembled. The steering committee is responsible for

- Implementing staff member and surgeon training
- Reviewing clinical cases
- Approving proctors
- Making decisions about the robotics program team.

The first task for the committee, however, is to set goals and develop a plan to accomplish them. Our perioperative director coordinated the program initiation and brought together the robotics steering committee, which consisted of facility administrators (eg, the chief financial officer, chief nursing officer, chief executive officer), surgeons, anesthesia care providers, a member of marketing services, and a robotic surgical system company representative. Steering committee members must ask questions such as

- Can a robotics program be successful in this community?
- How will a robotics program complement existing surgical programs?
- How will success be measured (eg, improved clinical outcomes, shorter hospital stays, higher procedure volume)?

The steering committee must establish a budget, and the facility should be prepared to make an initial investment of up to $2 million.[8] Financial representatives of the steering committee must take into account not only the initial investment but also ongoing maintenance, increased procedure costs, additional instrumentation and equipment, increased staff member educational needs and training costs, and marketing. After the budget is prepared, flexibility is needed until the program is well established.

The steering committee should establish a "beachhead" procedure in the initial kickoff. A beachhead procedure is one that can be extensively researched and is widely established in the robotics programs of other hospitals that incorporate the most current, evidence-based practices.[8] Robotic prostatectomy is often selected for the beachhead procedure at hospitals where a robotics program is being established. Focusing on one procedure in the development phase increases technical proficiency and provides the benchmark for other procedures down the road. With repetitive exposure, the team is then able to learn, lead, and successfully develop a surgical standard and clinical pathway for other procedures.

At our facility, approval was granted to purchase the da Vinci robotic surgical system, and it arrived in September 2008. Initially, the goal was for urologic surgeons to perform prostatectomies; however, gynecology and general surgery were soon added to the program. The gynecologists expressed an early interest in performing robotic hysterectomies, and this interest was accommodated. As a result of limited operating room time availability for the urologists, we began with 2 beachhead procedures (ie, robotic prostatectomy, robotic hysterectomy) and incorporated gynecology as well.

Education

Staff member education is the foundation for initiating any successful program. Education of the initial robotics team is a complex process involving all areas of the surgical department. Staff members who participate in the development of the robotics program should display a passionate interest and be leaders in their current practice. We learned that it is helpful to recruit an initial surgical team to train and gain competence with the new technology and beachhead procedure. The team members will gain the necessary knowledge and expertise to excel at the beachhead procedure, which lays the competency foundation for future staff member training. After the beachhead procedure is established, the team can begin incorporating more specialties to increase system usage and help distribute costs across departments. In our program development phase, we trained all lead staff members from 3 specialties: urology, gynecology, and general surgery. This proved cumbersome and inefficient, and there were many communication flaws. This experience supports the need to establish an initial surgical team to become competent with the one procedure and then pass the gained knowledge and experience on to subsequently trained staff members. Additional training also is needed for staff members in other supporting departments.

Many steps are involved in educating and training the surgical team. The education process starts weeks before the robot arrives in the surgical department. The surgeon starts by studying a CD-ROM provided by the robotics company representative and then completes an online examination. The surgeon then attends training at a practice facility, where he or she practices docking techniques and using the equipment. The surgeon then performs procedures with the robot on a pig in a laboratory. The surgeon practices dissection, ligation, and knot tying and also performs procedures such as hysterectomies and cystectomies. Immediately after training in the laboratory, the surgeon performs at least 2 procedures with a robotic proctor (ie, a board-certified surgeon with robotic training) and completes a total of 6 proctored procedures before performing robotic procedures independently.[9,10]

The circulating nurses, surgical technologists, and anesthesia care providers also are sent to observe robotic surgery at a nearby facility with an established robotic surgery program. The staff members are given an opportunity to observe and ask questions specific to the role they will perform. After the observation phase, education continues in the operating room with the robotic company representative. The company representative educates the initial team of nurses and surgical technologists on all of the electronics needed for robotic surgery and how to

- Connect the robotic system components
- Calibrate the robot for optimal use
- Troubleshoot technical problems that may arise during a procedure.

An important element of the education is what to do when an emergent situation arises and the procedure must be aborted. Staff members are instructed how to safely and quickly disconnect the robot (ie, detaching the robotic instruments from the trocars and then physically backing the patient cart away from the surgical field). Staff members practice procedure-specific techniques with the robotic representative.

After the initial training has been conducted and the robotic surgical team is comfortable with various robotic procedures, it is time to introduce additional staff members to the procedures and develop a set of competencies. **Table 1** is a set of competencies developed at St Joseph's Medical Center. These competencies are intended for the circulating nurse and the scrub person, whether that person is a nurse or surgical technologist. Although circulating nurses may not be responsible for performing instrument cleaning in some facilities, it is imperative that they understand the delicacy and mechanics of the instruments as well as the process to decontaminate and reprocess them.

Progress review should be conducted at regular robotics steering committee meetings. The strategy of the program should be analyzed and adjusted as needed to benefit the community, health care facility, and potential patient population. For instance, after 40 successful procedures were completed in 6 months, the steering committee recommended implementing a robotics coordinator. Success should be rewarded and major accomplishments, such as completing the 100th robotic procedure and increased public interest, should be made known to recognize growth, hard work, and dedication.

Robotics Coordinator

The robotics coordinator is a clinical expert and care coordinator for patients undergoing robotically assisted surgery. The robotics coordinator

- Orchestrates scheduling of robotic procedures
- Ensures instrument availability for robotic procedures
- Assists intraoperatively during robotic procedures
- Provides patient and staff member education
- Assists with research efforts and data collection.[5(p637)]

Table 2 outlines the duties and responsibilities of the robotics coordinator.

It is vital that the robotics coordinator actively participate in any robotic procedure that is performed at the facility. The robotics coordinator can act as a liaison

Table 1
Perioperative robotics competencies*

1. Arrange the robotic system in the operating room to maximize safety and ergonomic benefit:
   a. Components—positioning considerations
   b. Vision cart—moving and locking into place
   c. Patient cart—where and how to operate motor drive and lock wheels
   d. Surgeon console—moving and locking into place
2. Assemble all system connections
   a. AC connections to system components
   b. Camera head
   c. System cables
   d. Auxiliary connections
3. Start the system and establish homing (ie, allowing the machine to center itself after being turned on, which places the instrument, camera arms, and surgeon toggle controls in the optimal starting location)
   a. Vision cart
   b. Surgeon console
   c. Patient cart
4. Drape the system in sequence to maintain sterility
   a. Ports, instruments, and arm clutching
   b. Instrument arm
   c. Touch screen monitor and camera arm
   c. Endoscope and assembly
5. Set up the vision system
   a. White balance
   b. Endoscope assembly, calibration, and configuration
6. Set up the patient cart
   a. Patient cart docking
   b. Instrument arm docking (ie, insertion, withdrawal)
   c. Instrument cleaning both intraoperatively and postoperatively
7. Set up the surgeon console
   a. Left pod overview
   b. Footswitch panel overview
   c. Surgeon comfort settings
8. Identify safety features (ie, how to take proper action when recoverable and nonrecoverable faults occur)
   a. Error handling
   b. Recoverable fault
9. Perform the system shutdown procedure
   a. Shutdown preparation
   b. Drape removal
   c. Robotic arm stowage
   d. Power-down procedure
   e. Cleaning
   f. Storage and care

*Data from Intuitive Surgical® System Training: System Skill Practicum Participant's Guide. Sunnyvale, CA: Intuitive Surgical; 2009; and Wright D. The Ultimate Guide to Competency Assessment in Healthcare. 3rd ed. Minneapolis, MN: Creative Health Care Management; 2005.

between the staff members, surgeons, administrators, marketing team members, and the robotics company. Establishing this role is instrumental in the early phases of program development and, ideally, would be established at the onset of a new robotics program to ensure consistent goal setting and accomplishment, program evaluation, and provision of exceptional patient care.[5]

Table 2
Robotics coordinator responsibilities*

Clinical practice
- Act as a care coordinator
- Provide direct patient care
- Organize and maintain inventory of required robotic supplies and equipment
- Orchestrate the scheduling of procedures
- Provide clinical expertise

Education
- Orient and educate surgical staff members along with the perioperative educator
- Educate surgical patients and their family members
- Educate the general public and potential patients

Administration
- Act as a liaison in the health care facility
- Act as a liaison between the facility and the manufacturer and company representatives
- AAct as a liaison with the general public and other health care professionals outside the health care facility
- Act as a liaison between the facility and the manufacturer and company representatives

Research
- Participate in data gathering
- Participate in data management
- Ensure data dissemination

Professional
- Maintain clinical expertise and professional skills
- Participate in data management
- Develop and engage in leadership and consultant activities

*Data from Francis P. Evolution of robotics in surgery and implementing a perioperative robotics nurse specialist role. AORN J 2006;83(3):630–50.

Nursing Care of the Patient Undergoing a Robot-Assisted Surgery

The preoperative care and postoperative care are virtually the same for robotic procedures as they are for traditional laparoscopic procedures, and with both, patient education is a key component to recovery. There is potential for patient discharge the day after surgery, so instructions must begin before the patient undergoes the procedure. The words that nurses use to describe the surgical robot must be chosen carefully. Surgical team members must be aware that the term *robot* may cause feelings of anxiety or fear, especially if the patient has not been educated on the use of surgical robots. Unlike industrial robots, surgical robots are not autonomous or independent. It must be described as a tool used by the surgeon and not a device that acts independently or is preprogrammed.

The first robotic procedures performed at any hospital can prove lengthy and time consuming; for instance, initially a robotic prostatectomy may take up to 8 hours compared with an open prostatectomy, which takes approximately 2 hours. Research has shown that it takes surgeons 20 procedures before their operating times begin to decrease because the learning curve is steep.[2] Therefore, to promote positive outcomes, perioperative nurses should provide intraoperative warming measures and must be cautious with positioning.

Maintaining patient normothermia during a robotic procedure is important to prevent adverse consequences as a result of procedure length, especially in the initial procedures during which surgeons and staff members are still honing their skills. General anesthesia or major regional anesthesia impairs the thermoregulatory function of the body. While under anesthesia, the patient is unable to shiver and the patient's vessels do not vasoconstrict. Adverse consequences of hypothermia include increased incidence of postoperative surgical site infections, prolonged recovery and need for postanesthesia care, impaired medication metabolism, and increased risk of cardiac complications. Forced-air warming is an effective method of preventing unplanned hypothermia for patients who are anesthetized.[11,12]

Maintaining skin integrity must be at the forefront of patient preparations. Trendelenburg and lithotomy are common positions for robotic surgery. The surgeon may require that the stirrups and robotic arms be repositioned during a robotic procedure. If this occurs, the circulating nurse should reassess the patient each time the patient's position is changed or modified.[13] Sheer-related injuries are a risk of robotic surgery that should be prevented; securing the patient to the operating room bed with proper padding and movement-limiting devices can decrease the likeliness of this type of injury. Venous return can be decreased because of knee flexion, so using antiembolic stockings or intermittent compression devices is a requirement.

Concerns of the anesthesia care provider during robotic surgery include fluid shifts and restriction of respirations. The anesthesia care provider must carefully monitor fluid levels to prevent detrimental fluid shifts, which can increase blood pressure and intracranial pressure and cause facial edema, congestion, and atelectasis. Furthermore, the abdominal viscera can impede diaphragmatic movement and compress lung bases.

To provide safe care, the operating room requires highly trained personnel to operate, set up, and maintain the surgical robot. Perioperative nurses must be proficient in the setup, connections, and positioning of the robotic consoles. Nurses must have sufficient training in solving any mechanical problem so the surgeon can focus his or her complete attention on the procedure at hand. Nurses must be prepared for any emergent situation with proper supplies and knowledge of undocking procedures. The nurse must be knowledgeable about robotic instrumentation and understand how to load, unload, and clean all robotic instruments. Currently, at our facility, we are creating an intraoperative clinical pathway for nurses, both novice and experienced, who care for patients undergoing robotic surgery to ensure consistent patient care.

Troubleshooting

The robotic surgical system has the technology and capabilities of the most complex computer system in health care. It is able to store memory of past events and errors to the system as well as allow "live" interaction with technical engineers and support staff members from the headquarters of the robot company. In the event of a technical error, surgical team members can receive live technical support on the telephone from the engineers at the company. The actual system is connected through the Internet, which transmits all computerized messages to the engineers at company headquarters no matter where in the world the surgical team may be situated. This is comforting to the surgical team because in the event of a machine error or system fault, help is only a telephone call away. The engineers can log in and see what the surgical team members see on their monitors. The engineer can diagnose the problem and may even fix the problem from the headquarters location.[9]

To troubleshoot when a machine fault occurs during a procedure, the team must follow the instructions displayed on the monitors. There are 2 main faults that can occur: "recoverable" and "nonrecoverable." A recoverable fault occurs when there is either a technical or physical error problem with the machine. The classification *recoverable* means that the procedure can continue as normal after the team has identified and fixed the cause of the fault. The system has an alarm to alert the team of such faults, which includes a series of error beeps, messages on the monitors, and error light–emitting diode lights on the patient cart arms. The machine locks when a fault occurs and is easily unlocked when the problem has been identified. In rare instances, the machine will need to be undocked and restarted for the robotic procedure to continue.[9]

A nonrecoverable fault is one that occurs when the machine will no longer function in a safe manner, requiring the surgical team to abandon the technology and convert the procedure to another approach (eg, standard laparoscopy, open). For example, if the power goes out with no generator backup, the robotic approach will have to be aborted.

An emergency stop button is located on the surgeon console. There is also an emergency power-off button on the back of the surgeon console if the power needs to be completely shut off to the system for any emergent reason, such as a physical hazard in the operating room (eg, fire) or the need to convert to an open procedure because of an emergency such as internal hemorrhage. The system must be plugged into an appropriate outlet at all times. There is battery backup for the surgeon console and patient cart; however, the battery life is only 5 minutes.[9]

If a procedure needs to be converted from a robotic procedure to open surgery, the surgical team must take a few additional steps. The surgical team must remove the robotic instruments and endoscope from the patient, disconnect the robotic arms from the trocars, and undock the patient cart. The team can then proceed with the open procedure as a normal transition from laparoscopic to open surgery.

Marketing

The hospital marketing team or representative should actively inform the public of the hospital's new program to ensure its success. A surgical robotic program will not be successful if the robot is not used. One method is to develop a web site to educate the community and target audience. The robotics coordinator and team of staff members and surgeons should educate others at the facility (eg, employees, board members, referring physicians). This could take the form of an initial open house and display of the robotic system to promote understanding. Patient and physician education seminars could be held with the help of local media.

Promoting a robotic surgery program in larger cities can be simpler because of multiple opportunities for television, newsprint, billboard, and radio advertising. In a rural community, however, promoting a robotic surgery program is more challenging. In our community, for example, there is one public television network, which limits television advertising opportunities to public cable access. Also, there is only one local newspaper and only a couple of major roadways for billboard advertisements. The cost of advertising is greatly reduced, but the audience reached is limited.

For a small hospital, promoting a robotic surgical program is a must because of competition with large city programs. Unique marketing opportunities are available, however. Our vendor has five traveling robots that are used for promotional purposes to allow the public to see and touch the robots and ask questions. We have reserved robots from our vendor several times for public promotions. The first promotion for St Joseph's Medical Center was held at a local hotel, where a urologist gave an educational lecture on prostate surgery. The second promotion was held in the hospital lobby for patients and guests. We also conducted a media promotion with our own robot at the hospital with a local resident who is a national fishing television personality. He demonstrated the robot's ease of use by tying flies and baiting hooks. For the next promotion, we demonstrated one of the traveling robots at a local sporting goods store during an active weekend. The retailer allowed the robotic system to be set up at the store and provided a drawing for a $100 gift certificate. Future marketing plans include a public surgery open house to promote the robot and use of one of the traveling robots at a local minor league baseball game.

SUMMARY

Development of a surgical robotics program is intense. With a team of dedicated and educated professionals, however, a hospital has the potential to progress from good to great. No longer does the latest technology have to be confined to the major metropolitan areas. As it expands into the rural communities, smaller health care facilities can offer their patients the best option for minimally invasive surgery. Surgeons and staff members must strive to provide the best care in a rural community, and robotic surgery is in the forefront of this vision.

REFERENCES

1. Francis P, Winfield HN. Medical robotics: the impact on perioperative nursing practice. Urol Nurs 2006;26(2):99–108.
2. Berlinger N. Robotic surgery—squeezing into tight places. N Engl J Med 2006; 354(20):2099–101.
3. Franklin B. Robotic surgical systems. Biomed Instrum Technol 2006;40(6):461–4.
4. Francis P. Evolution of robotics in surgery and implementing a perioperative robotics nurse specialist role. AORN J 2006;83(3):630–50.
5. daVinci® Surgical System frequently asked questions: force feedback. IntuitiveSurgical.com. Available at: http://www.intuitivesurgical.com/corporate/newsroom/mediakit/da_Vinci_Surgical_System_FAQ.pdf. Accessed April 19, 2010.
6. Hagen ME, Meehan JJ, Inan I, et al. Visual clues act as a substitute for haptic feedback in robotic surgery. Surg Endosc 2008;22(6):1505–8.
7. Recommendations for building a da Vinci Robotic Surgery Program. Sunnyvale (CA): Intuitive Surgical, Inc; 2006.
8. Intuitive Surgical. da Vinci® Surgical System User's Manual. Sunnyvale (CA): Intuitive Surgical; 2007.
9. Haggag A. Robotic surgery: when technology meets surgical precision. Internet J Health 2006;5(1). Available at: http://www.ispub.com/ostia/index.php?xmlFilePath=journals/ijh/vol5n1/davinci.xml Accessed March 8, 2010.
10. Recommended practices for the prevention of unplanned perioperative hypothermia. In: Perioperative standards and recommended practices. Denver (CO): AORN, Inc; 2010. p. 298.
11. Hegarty J, Walsh E, Burton A, et al. Nurses' knowledge of inadvertent hypothermia. AORN J 2009;89(4):701–13.
12. Heizenroth PA. Positioning the patient for surgery. In: Rothrock J, editor. Alexander's Care of the patient in surgery. 13th edition. St Louis (MO): Elsevier; 2007. p. 149–50.

Role of the Perioperative Nurse in Robotic Surgery

Cynthia C. Thomas, BSN, RN, CNOR

KEYWORDS
- Robotic surgery • Gynecologic surgery
- Perioperative nursing care • Surgical robotics

AN EVOLUTION INTO PERIOPERATIVE NURSING

The ability to help shape the future is a rewarding opportunity for the perioperative nurse ready for a challenge. Robotics has given perioperative nurses the opportunity to adapt their practice, think creatively, and develop efficient clinical practices to care for their patient's safety. The prospect of developing a robotic surgery program can be quite overwhelming. Using the skills and knowledge of an experienced perioperative nurse will allow development of an efficient robotic program.

Medical advancements have continued to improve minimally invasive surgery (MIS). Performing surgery through smaller incisions with telescopes and long laparoscopic instruments eliminates the need for large incisions. Robotic assistance has become advantageous in the MIS arena.[1] Advantages for patients include shorter hospital stay, less pain, and decreased blood loss and cosmesis.[2] The benefits of robotic assistance have been magnified for the surgeon by improving dexterity, intuitive instrument management, 3D visualization, camera stability and control, surgeon ergonomics, 7 degree wrist action instruments, and independent activation of monopolar and bipolar energy.[3] These advancements are now allowing surgeons to offer MIS to a greater number of patients. Robotics has helped bridge the gap between laparotomy and MIS.

The patient today is more aware of new surgical technology regarding various surgical procedures. Accordingly, hospitals must determine how robotic surgery will best serve their patient population and identify surgeons who are interested in this technology. Such factors as equipment cost, training and credentialing physicians, adequate operating room space, and usage must be carefully evaluated.

STRATEGIES FOR BUILDING A STRONG ROBOTIC TEAM

Building a professional sports team requires money, a good head coach, and talented players.[4] This is also true when building a strong robotic program. The ideal team

Woman's Hospital, 9050 Airline Highway, Baton Rouge, LA 70815, USA
E-mail address: cynthia.thomas@womans.org

Perioperative Nursing Clinics 6 (2011) 227–234
doi:10.1016/j.cpen.2011.06.005
1556-7931/11/$ – see front matter © 2011 Elsevier Inc. All rights reserved.

Table 1
Robotic nurse coordinator job roles

Area of Practice	Specific Roles
Clinical practice	Acts as clinical coordinator Provides direct patient care Provides clinical expertise
Education	Orients and trains nursing personnel Trains and mentors health care students Liaison to lay public
Administration	Acts as liaison within institution Acts as liaison to manufacturer Acts as liaison outside institution with lay public and outside health care professionals
Research	Participates in data gathering Participates in data management
Professional	Maintains clinical expertise and skills Develops and engages in management and consultant con

includes surgeons, nurses, a surgical technologist, central processing personnel, an anesthesia provider, and operating room assistants. Each member brings his or her expertise to the program and develops his or her roles before, during, and after surgery.[3] As mentioned above, a multidisciplinary team is essential. The addition of a coordinator to facilitate the process can prove to be effective. By having each area represented within the team, it allows each member to contribute to the building of the team and the success of the program.

DEVELOPING ROLE OF THE PERIOPERATIVE NURSE ROBOTIC COORDINATOR

A perioperative nurse robotic coordinator is important for the start-up of a new robotic program. This nurse coordinator has expertise in MIS, which provides continuity to the robotic environment. Proficiency in MIS procedures transitions to the technology of robotics with ease. This nurse is already accustomed to the arena of high-tech equipment. Troubleshooting skills and the knowledge of patient care and safety are elements that contribute to critical thinking skills, which result in favorable surgical outcomes. The coordinator becomes the team's expert who focuses on the new technology. Team members use this knowledge and develop critical thinking skills to build the team's expertise. The coordinator also provides the necessary knowledge base to assist potential surgeons and team members by providing up-to-date information to promote the technology. The duties and responsibilities of the robotic nurse coordinator should include clinical practice, education, and research (**Table 1**).[5]

To achieve expertise, the nurse robotic coordinator can begin by observing robotic procedures and consulting existing robotic experts. Manufacturers' representatives offer coordinator programs to further educate nurses about the robotic system. These programs allow coordinators who are actively working in their institutions to network and share ideas. It is the robotic nurse coordinators who bear the responsibility to incorporate AORN standards of care,[6] attend continuing educational programs, network with colleagues, and review current literature. The robotic coordinator maintains clinical skills necessary to provide high-quality patient care in the operating room. Functioning clinically also allows the coordinator to assess the utilization of robotic equipment, instruments, and supplies.[5] This allows the nurse to understand

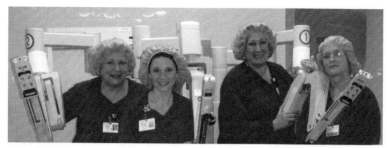

Fig. 1. Robotic Surgical Team.

and address staff members' suggestions and concerns. The robotic nurse coordinator will carry this education model back to the team she develops.

The educating role of the robotic coordinator includes orienting new team members, assuring competencies of team, assisting with educational opportunities for visiting and resident staff, and troubleshooting. Education and networking expands outside the institution via professional organizations, boards, and community outreach. This provides awareness for the hospitals and opportunities for promoting leading-edge medical care for the community.

PERIOPERATIVE TEAM

Perioperative planning should begin by identifying a core robotic team of 5 or 6 members. Robotic surgery requires 2 surgeons, a scrub nurse/technician, 2 circulating nurses, and an anesthesia provider. A dedicated team of surgeons and nurses is crucial to the successful implementation of robotics,[7] for it allows members to gain expertise, improve efficiency in set-up time, shortens procedure time, and facilitates turnover. As the initial team members gain confidence and experience, additional members can be added. Team members should have the following qualifications:

- Possess a high level of technical competency and understanding of equipment, its function, and troubleshooting.
- Be adaptive.
- Be willing to develop a new foundation to train future members.
- Be compatible with surgeons for ease of communication.
- Be flexible in scheduling to cover cases during early learning.
- Be self-motivated and positive.
- Be knowledgeable in MIS.
- Be knowledgeable in AORN standards of care.

Educating the team on the use of robotics in the operating room is critical. The robotic nurse coordinator will share her training experiences with the team. Visiting an institution with an existing program and allowing team members to visualize a team in action gives them the opportunity to interact with team members who share their same function. This approach allows brainstorming among team members and aids in the development of the hospital's individual program. Manufacturers' representatives are helpful in providing the robotic team with their expertise of the robotic system, but it is the perioperative nurse's role to implement standards of care for the patient in the area of safety, fluid and electrolyte balance, and sterility (**Fig. 1**). Team members will pool their knowledge to develop procedural standards.

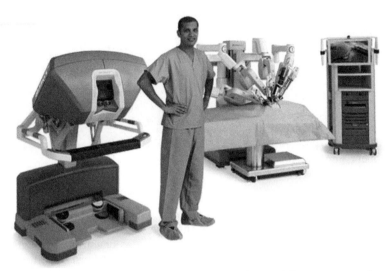

Fig. 2. The Robotic System consists of three pieces: (*left to right*) surgeon console, patient cart and vision tower.

Before the initial robotic procedure, a mock procedure will allow the team to be more efficient and review:

- Placement of equipment in the operating room
- Equipment operation
- Role playing for each team member
- Development of preference cards
- Organization of instrument sets
- Troubleshooting techniques.

ROBOTIC EQUIPMENT

MIS uses telescopes and long laparoscopic instruments through punctures in the patient's abdomen. The robotic system allows the surgeon to manipulate these instruments while sitting at the console that houses the master hand controls. The instrument's wristed movements are transferred via a computer to the patient via the robotic patient side cart. The robotic system is composed of 3 parts: patient-side cart, vision tower, and surgeon console (**Fig. 2**).[8]

The patient-side cart (robot slave unit) is positioned at the appropriate side of the patient depending on the procedure to be preformed. The surgeon places 3 or 4 sleeves into the patient's abdomen. The robotic arms are attached to these sleeves. The sleeves allow passage of robotic wristed instruments. The center arm holds the 3D camera and telescope. The left and right arms are used for the special endoscopic wristed instruments. A fourth arm is optional and can be positioned to the right or left side of the patient for retraction instruments.

The vision tower houses the touchscreen high-definition television, dual cameras, the camera merging system that provides the 3D image, focusing controls, and microphone switch. The touchscreen allows the nurse to open the computer software screen that aligns the 2 cameras with a telescope for the 3D image. The touchscreen also has telestration capabilities useful for teaching. The Tile Pro (Intuitive Surgical

Inc, Sunnyvale, CA, USA) feature allows the surgeon to input radiological data from ultrasound, CT, or MRI.

The surgeon console allows the surgeon to operate from a remote master controller with a combination of hand controls and foot pedals.[8] Pedals control the camera movement, camera focus, energy units, and clutching pedal, which allow for repositioning of hand controls that provides instrument range of motion. The surgeon console also contains buttons to power up the robotic system, change left and right orientation, and deactivate faults. The surgeon is capable of manipulating, repositioning, grasping, retracting, cutting, dissecting, coagulating, and suturing. A bedside assistant is still required for all robotic cases. They are responsible for instrument exchanges, suction, irrigation, suture introduction and retrieval, and additional retraction.[8] For gynecological cases, a cervical manipulator may be needed to provide counter traction by the surgical scrub.

OPERATING ROOM REQUIREMENTS AND EQUIPMENT PLACEMENT

The operating room should provide adequate space for equipment placement, room layout, availability of proper receptacles and circuits, imaging, internet access to broadcast to other facilities, and access to supplies. A dedicated room is optimal to avoid moving the system and risking damage to mechanical components.[7] The vision tower should be placed above the patient's right shoulder for the surgeon to view while obtaining initial pneumoperitoneum. Additional equipment can be placed on another cart next to the vision tower for the insufflator, irrigator, suction, electrical generator, and photographic equipment capability. The surgeon console should be placed opposite the vision tower to enable the surgeon to view the patient while seated. This position keeps the surgeon oriented to help direct his bedside assistants. The patient cart is positioned at the patient's foot or side depending on the procedure. Gynecological procedures use the patient cart with the patient positioned in lithotomy. As the program develops, equipment placement and instruments can be modified.

INSTRUMENTS AND SUPPLIES

Standardizing setups help streamline procedural needs and prevent opening unnecessary supplies.[5] Placement of setup pictures for staff to view will be beneficial for orienting new team members. Communication to the staff with use of preference cards contributes to efficiency and decreases turnover time.

Robotic instruments differ from laparoscopic instruments. They are reusable for a preset number of uses. This count is kept on a computer chip in each instrument. It is necessary for the team members to monitor these uses for proper disposal and reordering of instruments. The robotic coordinator and sterile processing manager should collaborate on proper trays and packaging of these supplies. Robotic instruments that are seldom used can be packaged separately and kept on the robotic surgery cart and opened as needed. The reusable instruments must be properly cleaned and sterilized according to the manufacturer's recommendations. Sterile processing staff should be oriented on these procedures (**Fig. 3**).

PERIOPERATIVE CARE OF THE ROBOTIC PATIENT

Perioperative care for the robotic patient is the same as any MIS procedure. Educating the staff on robotic procedures through in-service training will provide them with factual information to share with patients and families. Patients need to understand that the robot is a sophisticated tool that allows surgeons to perform procedures with a minimally invasive approach. This will improve patient satisfaction

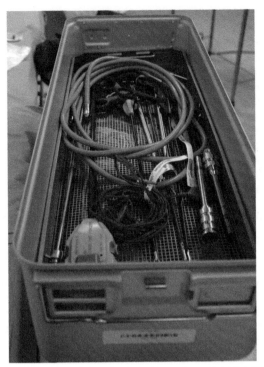

Fig. 3. Robotic instruments are sterilized in a container for easy accessibility.

in knowing that their nurse is knowledgeable about their surgery. Additional patient preoperative teaching should be added to alleviate fear of the robotic procedure.[1] MIS has shortened the patient's postoperative stay, therefore postoperative education should be addressed early. Educating the patient on postoperative expectations may decrease preoperative stress.

Intraoperavively, the perioperative nurse and team prepare for the surgery. The beginning of a robotic program involves the team planning and managing their time wisely. The learning curve for the team should be considered. Allowing for additional time in setting up and performing the procedures is recommended. These times will shorten as the team gains experience and skill. Team members need to be patient and share ideas to improve and become proficient. These ideas should be shared and reviewed at post-procedural meetings. The members of the team should be open to change and not mind enduring the growing pains of implementing a new program. See **Table 2** for procedural competencies.

Standards of care for postoperative robotic MIS patients are the same as for the conventional MIS patient. Postoperative care should be tailored to the patient's specific needs and expected surgical outcomes. Studies report that patients who had robotic surgery have decreased postoperative pain, and therefore require minimal pain medication.[2] Preoperative nausea protocols minimize postoperative nausea. Patients frequently have earlier discharge, decreasing the amount of time for patient education. This increases the responsibility preoperative nurses have in patient education. Earlier discharge places an additional responsibility on patients and their home care attendant. Providing written postoperative care instructions for the caregiver decreases feelings of anxiety before discharge.

Table 2
Robotics surgical system staff member competency
Purpose
The purpose of the robotic surgical system competency is to validate the ability to perform/respond to required competencies in using the robotic system.
Critical Elements
Describe moving all 3 robotic components before and after procedures.
Demonstrate plugging in all electrical parts of robotic system appropriately.
Demonstrate connecting 3 components of robotic system to each other.
Power up system and demonstrate correct "homing" procedure.
Fold robotic arm cart in a manner that protects the system.
Correctly power down system after verifying instrument use.
Instrumentation
Correctly input camera and alignment into system.
Demonstrate proper draping of surgical arm cart and telescope/camera.
Successfully complete calibration of telescopes
Verbally identify each robotic instrument.
Demonstrate proper placement and removal of robotic instruments.
Verbalize correct interpretation of robotic icons on monitor.
Identifies location of emergency wrench
Identifies application of use
Verbalizes emergency situation of power loss or nonrecoverable faults
Verbalizes correct action for recoverable faults
Identifies location of emergency resources in case of malfunction
Properly drives and positions system for procedure
Properly removes system after procedure including undraping
Identifies instrument "lives" on monitor and disposes of as needed
Properly undrapes telescope/camera and stores cords

POST-PROCEDURAL EVALUATION

Monitoring outcomes and success of a robotic program should be implemented by specifying measurable objectives for caseload baselines. Some outcomes to measure specifically are procedure times, blood losses, analgesic postoperative requirements, length of stay, patient satisfaction, and follow-up. Performance over time using benchmarks for complications, average length of stay, and cost per case may also be evaluated. Outcomes of this data should be shared with staff and used to better patient care. Staff improvements and procedural changes that improve staff performance will provide patients with a continued high level of care.

SUMMARY

As advancements in MIS are developed, more patients will be given the opportunity of having an MIS procedure. Perioperative nurses must work hard to educate and train themselves on all new technology that enters our workplace while at the same time recognizing and seizing the opportunities that lie ahead.[1] Adhering to basic nursing practices enables the nurse to retain the human side of caring but with the advanced knowledge necessary to ensure a successful outcome from MIS procedures. As perioperative nurses, we can redirect our patient focus in this high-performance, automated, and sometimes cold world of technology by focusing on solid nursing principles.

REFERENCES

1. Francis P, Winfield H. Medical robotics: the impact on perioperative nursing practice. Urol Nurs 2006;26:99–108.
2. Chen C, Falcon T. Robotic gynecologic surgery: past, present, and future. Clin Obstet Gynecol 2009;52:335–43.
3. Mendivil A, Holloway R, Boggess JF. Emergence of robotic assisted surgery in gynecologic oncology: American perspective. Gynecol Oncol 2009;114:524–31.
4. Tabor W. Robotic surgery. Nursing 2007;37:48–50.
5. Conner R. Perioperative standards and recommended practices. 2010 edition. Association of Operative Room Nurses (AORN); 2010.
6. Francis P. Evolution of robotics in surgery and implementing a perioperative robotics nurse program. AORN J 2006;83:630–42, 644–6, 649–50.
7. Steers W, LeBeau S, Cardella J, et al. Establishing a robotic program. Urol Clin North Am 2004;31:773–80.
8. Visco A, Advincula A. Robotic gynecologic surgery. Obstet Gynecol 2008;112: 1369–83.

Patient Advocacy in Robotic Surgery

Christina G. Thell, RN, BSN, CNOR

KEYWORDS
- Patient advocacy • Robotic surgery • Perioperative care
- Patient anxiety

Although robotic surgery can be an exciting addition to a surgeon's practice and a hospital's repertoire of procedures offered to the community, it brings a lot of apprehension for some patients. For many patients, new technology seems a bit scary as they wonder, "Am I the first patient this is being used on? Is this still an experiment? Is the machine going to fail? Why isn't the surgeon going to operate on me?" These are the questions that must be cleared up in the beginning, and we, the medical community, must not forget that patients see new technology in a completely different way than we do. It is our job to educate them on the correct purpose and function of robotic technology so that they may overcome this apprehension and anxiety. "Although other health professionals advocate for their patients or clients, nursing has designated the advocate role as a central role of nursing practice."[1]

PERIOPERATIVE NURSING AND PATIENT ADVOCACY

AORN states, "The perioperative RN, through professional and patient-centered expertise, is the primary patient advocate in the operating room and is responsible for monitoring all aspects of the patient's condition . . . During surgery, most patients are anesthetized or sedated and are powerless to make decisions on their own behalf. By employing their critical thinking, assessment, diagnosing, outcome identification, planning, and evaluation skills, the RN circulator directs the nursing care and coordinates activities of the surgical team for the benefit of the patient whose protective reflexes or self-care abilities are compromised by the procedure." It is this concept of patient advocacy that serves as the foundation of our care in the surgical arena. There is much literature that states the importance of this concept throughout the intraoperative environment, not only for legality and safety reasons, but also for driving patient outcomes. It has been proven that when a nurse advocates for a particular patient throughout their entire surgical experience, surgical outcomes are significantly improved.[2-4]

This concept of patient advocacy encompasses the whole of what it means to be a perioperative nurse. In an article written by Snowball, the author states that nurses

St. Joseph's Medical Center, 523 North 3rd Street, Brainerd, MN 56401, USA
E-mail address: cgthell@gmail.com.

Perioperative Nursing Clinics 6 (2011) 235–240
doi:10.1016/j.cpen.2011.05.001
1556-7931/11/$ – see front matter © 2011 Elsevier Inc. All rights reserved.

must embrace the role of decisional counselor so that patients may be offered the maximum amount of knowledge about their diagnosis and treatment options.[3] Establishing a therapeutic relationship in the preoperative phase allows us to educate patients so that they make an appropriate decision about their course. Snowball mentions that a number of patients "expressed sentiments about [the nurse] sharing a common humanity with patients and describe the need for the nurse to relate to people generally and for investing much of your human self in the relationship." Patients appreciate our openness and honesty with them, and establishing that trust and rapport eliminates the uncomfortable barrier that exists at times between the general public and medical staff.

It is important for patients to first understand us. This includes what their diagnosis means and what surgical and nonsurgical options are available to them. It is helpful to review why physicians make certain suggestions and what they mean. Also, ultimately, it is about patients making an informed decision and the right choice for them and their families. If we want patients to truly have informed consent for their procedure, all of these questions must be answered and understood. We must be aware that when the patient gives us their informed consent, it helps in maintaining their autonomy.[5]

It also is important for us to understand our patients. This begins with their medical and surgical history, of course. A thorough history will give us clues into their potential level of understanding and anxiety related to surgical procedures. Including their spiritual and cultural beliefs in our interview is vital in establishing empathy and to understand why they are making the choices they are. If the patient so desires, it may be helpful to include the family. Asking about the patient's level of education will help determine how to educate them so they understand the information. We must also determine how much information to give them. In an article written by Pritchard, it is suggested that "increasing the patient's knowledge of the forthcoming surgery may reduce his or her anxiety levels, but not all patients would respond positively to such information, and in some cases information provided no benefit."[6]

Reviewing all of this information in the preoperative environment, weeks before the proposed procedure, allows that nurse-patient relationship to form and knowledge to be passed on. This may happen over the phone or in the clinic but serves as the beginning of our advocacy role. As we have listened to our patients' wishes or requests, fears, confidences, religious and ethical issues, and so forth, we can use our judgment and expertise to pass this information on to the operating team to promote the best outcome for the patient.[4] This advocacy role can then be applied to the immediate preoperative and intraoperative phases, where the decisions we make as nurses have a direct correlation to the patient's surgical outcome. Let us not forget that advocacy "underscores the perioperative nurse's acts in informing and supporting patients they care for and taking action to achieve goals on behalf of those patients."[7]

PERCEPTIONS OF ROBOTIC TECHNOLOGY

Patient perceptions of robotic technology vary dramatically from science fiction to accurate reality. Understanding what previous comprehension the patient has of robotics can easily provide a starting point in accurate education. Patients may fall into one of three levels of understanding about robotic technology: ill-educated, some understanding, and clear understanding. Patients who are ill-educated may have no knowledge that this technology even exists; the concept may seem like something out of science-fiction movies to them. Patients who have completely inaccurate information about robotics would also fall into this category. Some patients believe that there is no surgeon at all, that the robot performs the procedure and is autonomous. Some believe that the machine has a mind of its own and is preprogrammed with the surgery to perform.

Patients who have some understanding may just need some clarification. They may have obtained their information through the internet, news programs, or word of mouth. Those who seem excited about this new technology seem to view it as a positive improvement for surgical procedures. Oftentimes, these individuals ask, "Am I a candidate for robotic surgery?" However, there are those who view it negatively, display much more apprehension about it, and usually are misinformed. At times it may take more work from the medical and nursing staff to change their preconceived notions.

Then there are the patients who have a clear understanding of robotic surgery. In an article written by Borch and colleagues[8] one of their patients "chose to undergo laparoscopic robotic prostatectomy because this was a less invasive procedure; and would theoretically give him a shorter recovery time." They also found that "with the increased use of the internet, patients were more informed. They seek out the latest techniques and are willing to travel in order to receive care from those urologists who offer this newest technology."[8] These individuals are usually patients or family members who have undergone robotic procedures; surgery staff or family of surgery staff; and those who are preparing to undergo a procedure in the near future. They have accurate information and a complete understanding, and are well educated on robotic surgery. Patients who have a clear understanding do very well with public relations. It can be quite beneficial to have them educating their family and peers with accurate information regarding robotic technology.

No matter what a patient's perception may be of robotic surgery, it is our job to clear up false information and educate our patients. Using layman's terms and describing the robotic technology as a tool is a great first step. The more accurate information we can spread throughout our patient population and community, the less apprehension and fear patients may come in with. When their doctor recommends robotic surgery, they will understand what is being suggested. We must be sensitive to patient's feelings about robotics. As anxiety affects our patients' postoperative outcomes, we must help them feel comfortable with this technology.

Although procedural information is important and necessary to promote a patient's understanding of robotics, an interesting concept of surgical education was detailed in an older article, which discussed the difference between procedural instruction and sensory instruction.[9] "Traditionally, in procedural instruction, you tell the patient the details of the procedure that is about to be performed . . . The perspective is that of the health professional delivering the care . . . In sensory instruction, you tell the patient the sights, sounds, odors, tastes, and feelings he can expect to experience . . . The perspective is that of the patient receiving the care."[9] Although this idea was brought forth in 1977, it is still applicable today with new technology. The authors found that preparing patients for the sensations they will experience decreased their level of distress and the fear associated with the surgical procedure, and "the more closely the experienced sensations reflect the expectations, the lower degree of distress."[9] For patients undergoing robotic surgery, we could include this sensory information along with the procedural information by telling them what they will see when they enter the operating room, what they may smell and taste during induction of anesthesia, the noises they may hear as they drift off, and the touches they may feel. It is believed that procedural information is best aimed for the less anxious patient and that sensory information is best for the more nervous patient.[10]

As the patient advocate, we have the responsibility to help our patients gain inner strength in order to control and conquer their fears.[11] We must be aware that the words we use, such as "robot," can spark feelings of uncertainty. Patients link the word robot to science fiction and an object completely mechanical with a mind of its own. Words such as "technology" or "tool" seem to bring less fear, and we must always be cognizant of what the patient may perceive as negative or frightening. Anxiety can stem from feelings of insecurity while being in an unfamiliar environment. Couple that with unfamiliar technology and major surgery and we can understand why patients hesitate at the idea of robotic surgery.

When educating our patients we must approach the topic with a sound understanding ourselves. If we are unsure of ourselves or the equipment we are using, then the patient will sense that. Any staff participating in robotic surgery should have a clear understanding of what and how it works.

Sometimes in all of our excitement of this new technology, we, nurses and doctors, may talk so highly of robotics that it portrays unrealistic expectations of the procedure and outcomes, though unintentional. Patients who get caught up in the hype and hope of robotic surgery may come into their procedure with these unrealistic expectations, such as returning to work in a week or two, not having any pain, and being able to mow the lawn only a few days after surgery. Although these stories are true, they are not the norm. It is our job to clear up these unrealistic expectations and convey the message that this is major surgery, even though it may not look like or feel like it. Patients who push themselves too far postoperatively will ultimately have a far longer recovery period than those who listen to their doctor, nurses, and their own bodies.

COMBINING PATIENT ADVOCACY WITH ROBOTIC TECHNOLOGY

As the patient prepares for his or her upcoming procedure, it is helpful to initiate a sound nurse-patient relationship early on. If a robotic coordinator has been established this would be an example of one of their roles. Allowing patients to ask plenty of questions will help maintain their autonomy and control over what is happening to them. Conducting an over-the-phone interview may be the first step in showing genuine interest in their well-being, which is necessary for true advocacy. Obtaining a sound medical and surgical history from them as well as their cultural and spiritual beliefs will aid in counseling their decisions about their care. Including the financial cost of the procedure and helping them in the approval process with their insurance company would also help ease a patient's trepidation over robotic surgery.

Facilitating a hospitable environment on arrival and a comfortable preoperative holding room will provide a warm welcome for the day of surgery. It has been suggested that music has the ability to relieve much of the fear and anxiety associated with facing the unknown,[12] so having some cheerful noise overhead may lighten the concern in the air. A friendly hello from the nurse who performed the preoperative preparation would also be appropriate at this point. This would allow time for further questions and discussion with the patient and family. In all, it is a time when the nurse can foster the trusting relationship with his or her patient so that the patient may feel comfortable with that nurse as an advocate. Maintaining their dignity throughout their surgical course begins as patients step into the well-known surgical gown. Giving patients privacy and letting them hold on to their modesty may also decrease their feelings of undue fear and anxiety.[10]

As it is time for the patient to make his or her way to the operating room, the nurse should remain with the patient at all times. Upon entering the room, it is comforting for the patient to be introduced to the team members as well as announcing the patient's wishes for what is to come. As their advocate we should give them "the opportunity to meet the members of their health care team so they can educate team members about the patient's expectations of the surgical process."[13] If the nurse determines that the patient is quite comfortable with the robotic technology, he or she should point it out to the patient. Describe the function of the machine such as, "that is the patient cart that moves the instruments the surgeon will use," "that is the camera that will allow us to see inside," and so forth. The nurse should provide a quiet and comfortable environment as the patient is drifting off.

Because the advocate relationship is the most vital role we play as circulating nurses, adhere to it. Do not leave the patient's side during induction of anesthesia because this can be a time of great fear and anxiety. Providing a gentle touch may reassure patients that you are still there, even when their eyes are closed. Once asleep, maintain their modesty until the last minute. We must remember what we would feel like laying on the table wearing only a gown. How would we want to be covered?

The intraoperative advocate role continues as we position the patient for the procedure. It is our job to keep the patient safe and free from injury. During robotic procedures, oftentimes the rest of the surgical team is quite focused on the procedure at hand and anesthesia is busy handling the challenges of steep Trendelenburg, and so forth. Therefore, the circulating nurse must keep a watchful eye on the rest of the patient beneath the drapes. Are they sliding or slipping? Are the robotic arms touching their legs or other part of their body? In the beginning of implementing robotic procedures, the need for a second circulator may be evident because of the complicatedness of the technology. There should always be a nurse focused solely on the patient, not on the technology or missing supplies. Until things become routine, a second circulating nurse should fill that role.

Once the procedure is finished, we continue our advocate role by making the patient presentable. Before patients leave the operating room, they should be clean and acceptable for the family to see. Provide a warm blanket for comfort and be by their side during emergence from anesthesia. They will be happy to see a familiar face and hear a familiar voice during wake up. Maintain a calm and quiet environment that promotes sleep to enhance their positive experience. Also, give a thorough report to the recovery room nurse. Patient advocacy during robotic surgery can be filled by more than one nurse. Perhaps the preoperative and postoperative advocacy role is filled by the robotic coordinator, while the intraoperative role is filled by a circulating nurse because the robotic coordinator may not be able to be in on the procedure. To maintain consistent advocacy, however, the initial nurse should have a positive relationship with the receiving nurse and display this to the patient during the introduction of a new advocate. One common topic of conversation is that of robotic procedure turnover time. Do not let the pressure of decreasing turnover time inhibit your ability to prepare the next patient for his or her procedure. "Perioperative nurses need time to make sure that individual patients are prepared for what may be a terrifying experience,"[13] and our role of patient advocate encompasses this belief.

Postoperatively, continue with the relationship that has been established by following up on the patient's experience and care. Be a liaison with the family, answer further questions, and provide encouragement during recovery. Postoperative phone calls are a wonderful way to finalize the patient advocate role. Follow up on how the patient is doing, inquire about his or her experience, and make necessary referrals if needed.

In conclusion, patient advocacy during robotic surgery is vital for the success of patients' outcomes. Establishing a trusting and positive nurse-patient relationship decreases the patient's fear and apprehension over surgery and this new technology.

Although much of the content in this article is subjective, it paves the way for further research. Literature regarding patient anxiety related to robotic surgery could not be found. A study may prove helpful in recognizing the triggers of patient anxiety and interventions for the patient advocate to provide more comfort.

REFERENCES

1. Hanks RG. The medical-surgical nurse perspective of advocate role. Nurs Forum 2010;45(2):97–107.
2. Perioperative nursing: court discusses standard of care. Legal Eagle Eye Newsletter Nurs Prof 2007;15(9):7–7.
3. Snowball J. Asking nurses about advocating for patients: "reactive" and "proactive" accounts. J Adv Nurs 1996;24(1):67–75.
4. Shewchuk M. Why a registered nurse (RN) in the OR? Can Oper Room Nurs J 2007;25(4):38.
5. Scott PA, Taylor A, Välimäki M, et al. Clinical practice. Autonomy, privacy and informed consent 4: surgical perspective. Br J Nurs 2003;12(5):311–9.
6. Pritchard MJ. Identifying and assessing anxiety in pre-operative patients. Nurs Stand 2009;23(51):35–40.
7. Boyle HJ. Patient advocacy in the perioperative setting. AORN J 2005;82(2):250–62.
8. Borch M, Hattala P, Baron B, et al. Laparoscopic radical robotic prostatectomy: a case study. Urol Nurs 2007;27(2):141–3.
9. A better way to calm the patient who fears the worst . . . patient-teaching technique. RN 1977;40:47–54.
10. Walker JA. Emotional and psychological preoperative preparation in adults. Br J Nurs 2002;11(8):567–75.
11. Petty C. A physicians' perspective on allaying patient's fears. AORN J 1985;41(3): 537,540,542.
12. Stevens K. Patients' perceptions of music during surgery. J Adv Nurs 1990;15(9): 1045–51.
13. Duffy WJ. President's message. Keeping surgical procedure turnover in perspective. AORN J 2004;80(4):637.

Robotic Surgery in Urology

Phillip Mucksavage, MD[a], David S. Chou, MD[b],*

KEYWORDS
- Robotics • Urology • Prostatectomy • Nephrectomy
- Complications • Outcome

Since the introduction of the da Vinci Surgical Robot System (Intuitive Surgical, Sunnyvale, CA, USA) in 1999, urologists have been at the forefront in the development and adoption of robotic surgery. Over the last year approximately 200,000 surgical operations have been performed using the da Vinci robotic surgical system, with more than 1000 robots now available throughout the United States.[1] It is estimated that more than 80% of all radical prostatectomies will be performed using robotic assistance in the upcoming year, while robot-assisted renal and bladder surgery volumes continue to increase.[2–7] Despite the costs to acquire, maintain, and operate the platform, it has gained widespread acceptance as an alternative to many laparoscopic and open surgical procedures.

The development of the surgical robot is an integral part in the evolution of minimally invasive surgeries, especially in urology. Minimally invasive surgeries offer the advantages of smaller incisions, shorter hospitalization, and faster recovery with equivalent outcomes to open surgeries.[8,9] However, traditional laparoscopic surgeries have severe limitations in the visual field, manual dexterity, precision, and ergonomics. These are particularly pronounced in complicated urologic surgeries in which delicate tissue handling, meticulous dissection, and precise reconstructions are essential. The current da Vinci robotic system combines the benefits of minimally invasive surgery with improved 3D visualization, enhanced dexterity, 7 degrees of instrument freedom, tremor reduction, and motion scaling.[10–12] This is all possible through an ergonomic and easy-to-control surgical console. With the aid of the da Vinci Surgical system, it became possible for traditional "open" surgeons to make the transition to "robot-assisted laparoscopic" surgeons.[13,14] As more urologic surgeons make this transition, robot-assisted laparoscopic radical prostatectomies (RALRP) have become the dominant surgical approach in the United States.

There are various issues that are unique to robotic surgery in urology. Because the RALRP is one of the most commonly performed robotic surgeries and the most common urologic operation, we will cover the preoperative, anesthesia, perioperative, and postoperative considerations associated with this operation. We will also focus

[a] University of California Irvine Medical Center, Orange, CA, USA
[b] Pacific Urology, Inc, Honolulu, Hawaii
* Corresponding author. 1029 Kapahulu Avenue, Suite 306, Honolulu, HI 96816.
E-mail address: admin@pacificuro.com

Perioperative Nursing Clinics 6 (2011) 241–258
doi:10.1016/j.cpen.2011.05.003

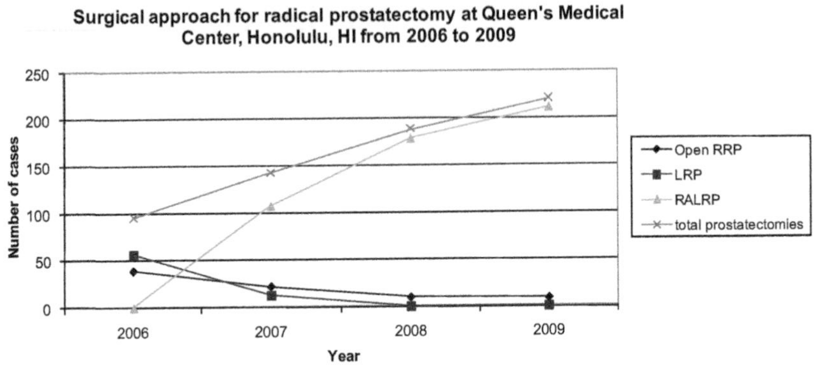

Surgical approach for radical prostatectomy at Queen's Medical Center, Honolulu, HI from 2006 to 2009

Fig. 1. Radical prostatectomies according to approach performed at Queen's Medical Center since the introduction of the da Vinci Surgical System.

on robot-assisted laparoscopic renal surgery, which is becoming more common and has many unique differences from a RALRP.

ROBOT PROSTATECTOMIES

Excluding skin cancer, prostate cancer is the most commonly diagnosed cancer among men in the United States and the second most common cause of cancer death among men.[15,16] It is a diagnosis made often from prostate biopsy, performed because of elevated levels of prostate-specific antigen (PSA) or an abnormal prostate on examination, or from transurethral resection of prostate. The decision for screening and treatment for prostate cancer is a highly individualized choice, and the controversies regarding screening or treatment for prostate cancer are beyond the scopes of the article. Once prostate cancer has been diagnosed, the treatment of the prostate cancer depends on the patient's age, overall medical condition, PSA level at the time of diagnosis, the Gleason score, and whether the cancer is localized within the prostate.

Standard treatments for localized prostate include active surveillance, radiation, radical prostatectomies, or cryotherapy. Any treatment for prostate cancer can greatly affect the patient's quality of life, carrying differing degrees of risks of urinary problems, bowel problems, sexual side effects, and incomplete treatment for the cancer. Surgical options for prostate cancer treatment include open retropubic radical prostatectomy (RRP), perineal radical prostatectomy, laparoscopic radical prostatectomy (LRP), and RALRP with the da Vinci Surgical System. Radical prostatectomy involves the removal of the prostate with its attached seminal vesicles and the ampulla of the vas. Because of real and perceived benefit, as well as market force, RALRP has become the dominant surgical approach.[14] It has been estimated that in 2010, 80% of all radical prostatectomies performed in the United States are done with robot assistance.[1] At the Queen's Medical Center in Honolulu, Hawaii, 96% of all radical prostatectomies performed in 2009 were done with the da Vinci Surgical System, with a marked decline in open and laparoscopic prostatectomies (**Fig. 1**).

Whether RALRP is superior to other surgical approaches is still a matter of debate. RALRP is still a relatively new treatment for prostate cancer, with most early published reports consisting of descriptions of the surgical techniques and short-term outcomes and safety data to support the feasibility of this approach. As the data mature, there are more long-term results showing the benefits and the drawbacks of RALRP. Even though the robotic technology offers advantages in greater precision and better visualization, there is no definitive evidence that these advantages translate into superior surgical outcome. The current data appear to show that RALRP offers similar functional and cancer control outcomes comparable with other surgical approaches, while offering the short-term advantages of decreased blood loss and faster recovery.[17–20]

PATIENT SELECTION

In general, patients who are candidates for open RRP are candidates for RALRP. Relative contraindications may include prior abdominal surgeries, obesity, severely enlarged prostate size, large median lobe, and pulmonary disease.

PREOPERATIVE DETAILS

Once a patient has been appropriately counseled regarding prostate cancer treatment options, and the patient has decided to proceed with RALRP, the patient is referred to his primary care physician or anesthesia preoperative evaluation center to undergo a preoperative medical evaluation. This may include a complete medical evaluation of the patient's cardiopulmonary, renal function, liver function, and hematologic status. Patients are also counseled to start performing Kegel exercises before surgery, and the option for a consultation with a physical therapist is offered to help the patient initiate pelvic floor exercise routines and to become familiarized with incontinence care products. The patients are encouraged to continue pelvic floor exercises after the surgery, with or without continued guidance from physical therapists.

The patients are counseled extensively on the details of the RALRP. The indications for pelvic lymph node dissection are discussed with the patient. The patients are counseled on what to expect on the day of the surgery, the hospital stay, and typical recovery course. The short- and long-term risks of the procedure are discussed in detail, and an operative consent form is reviewed and signed by the patient. The patient's medications are reviewed, and anticoagulants such as aspirin, clopidogrel, warfarin, and other nonsteroidal antiinflammatory drugs are stopped 1 week before the surgery. Heparin or enoxaparin can be used as bridge in patients at high risk. Over-the-counter vitamins and other supplements are also stopped 1 week before surgery. In general, the patients may continue with all of their other medications up to the day of the surgery.

The patient's sexual function is reviewed with the patient in detail. Depending on the patient's Gleason score, PSA, and estimate of the cancer volume on the biopsy, patients are counseled on unilateral, bilateral, or non-nerve–sparing procedures. The patients are counseled regarding the expected decline in their erectile functions postoperatively, which may take up to 2 years to recover, and also the possibility of shortening in penile length. In the recent literature, there has been support for the use of phosphodiesterase type 5 (PDE-5) inhibitors preoperatively for theoretical protective effects on erectile functions.[21] Therefore patients who are candidates for nerve-sparing RALRP are started 1 week before the surgery on low-dose sildenafil (Viagra) 25 mg once daily, vardenafil (Levitra) 5 mg once daily, or tadalafil (Cialis) 5 mg once daily. The patients also receive counseling regarding penile rehabilitation after the surgery. The options of staying on the PDE-5 inhibitors or using a vacuum-assisted device, intraurethral suppositories, or intracorporeal injection of vasoactive medications are discussed with the patients.[21,22] Usually, the preoperative PDE-5 inhibitors are continued on a twice weekly basis after the surgery.

Recently, more attention has been directed at possible adverse effects on vision from increased intraocular pressure from intraoperative Trendelenburg positioning.[23] Therefore, it may be important to obtain specific history regarding glaucoma or preoperative visual problems, and make appropriate referrals to an ophthalmologist preoperatively for evaluation.

Even though a full bowel preparation for RALRP has been described, a limited bowel preparation with a clear liquid diet 1 day before surgery and drinking 1 bottle of magnesium citrate the night before surgery has been adequate. The patient is instructed not to eat or drink anything after midnight, and they may take their medications as directed with a small sip of water on the morning of the surgery.

INTRAOPERATIVE CONSIDERATIONS

The patient is taken to the operating room. A time-out is taken to identify the patient and the procedure being performed. Antibiotic coverage generally includes cephazolin 1 g administered intravenously 30 minutes before the incision. Some surgeons also cover anaerobic bacteria with a dose of gentamycin 80 mg. Other appropriate alternative antibiotics are administered in patients with drug allergies to the standard prophylactic antibiotics. The patient is placed in a supine position, and bilateral lower extremity sequential compression stockings are placed. The patient is then placed under general endotracheal anesthesia. Invasive monitoring is not required for routine cases.

Positioning

Properly positioning of the patient begins before the patient enters the room. Poor planning and improper positioning can delay the procedure or lead to serious injuries. After the anesthesia team indicates that the patient is ready for positioning, the patient is placed on the table with the hip joints at the break in the bed. The upper limbs are then placed at his sides and tucked with bed sheets or plastic sleds. Each arm is generously padded and care is taken to ensure the hand is rotated so the thumb is facing up. This will limit the chance of neural injury. Because the robot is positioned and docked in between the patient's leg, either "leg spreaders" or cushioned "sharkfin" stirrups are used to place the patient in a modified lithotomy position. Care is taken that patient's hip joint lines up with the break of the leg rest if "leg spreaders" are used to avoid potential neuropathy.

The patient is then placed in a very steep Trendelenburg position. This allows for the bowel contents to move out of the pelvis and gives access to the bladder and prostate. "Egg crate" foams secured to the table using wide cloth tape keep the patient from sliding back while in the Trendelenburg position. Cross chest bindings have also been used when egg crates are not available, but egg crate padding is the easiest and most effective method to reduce sliding. Shoulder braces to hold the patient in place are not recommended because of risks of brachial plexus injury.[24]

Anesthesia Considerations

The use of nitric oxide during anesthesia is not recommended because of the risks of bowel distention that may interfere with the surgery.[25] Once the patient is under anesthesia, his eyelids are securely closed with tape to protect the his eyes. We also use protective goggles that remain on the patient for up to 1 hour after the operation to reduce patient and/or iatrogenic eye injury. Warming blankets are also used to prevent hypothermia.

Table 1
Physiological effects of pnuemoperitoneum in the Trendelenburg position

Cardiovascular system	↑ Systemic vascular resistance
	↑ Mean arterial pressure
	↑ Myocardial oxygen consumption
	↓ Renal, portal, and splenic flow
Respiratory system	↑ Ventilation-perfusion mismatch
	↓ Pulmonary compliance
	↑ Peak airway pressure
	↓ Functional residual capacity
	Pulmonary congestion and edema
	Hypercarbia, respiratory acidosis
Central nervous system	↑ Intracranial pressure
	↑ Cerebral blood flow
	↑ Intraocular pressure
Endocrine system	↑ Catacholamine release
	Activation of renin-angiotensin system
Others	Gastroesophageal regurgitation
	Venous air embolism
	Neuropraxia-brachial, perineal
	Facial and airway edema

When the patient is placed in the steep Trendelenburg position, there are a number of factors that must be considered. The Trendelenburg positioning along with the CO_2 pneumoperitoneum leads to significant changes in cardiovascular, cerebrovascular, and respiratory parameters (**Table 1**).[26,27] The anesthesiologist and nursing team in the room must be aware for the potential changes in cardiac and pulmonary parameters and be ready adjust the patient's positioning or reduce the pneumoperitoneum if necessary. Despite these considerable physiologic changes, multiple studies have demonstrated that they are well tolerated and not likely to lead to long-term adverse effects.[26,28] However, the procedure may take up to 2 to 4 hours or longer, and a vast list of complications ranging from edema to severe neurologic injuries, including loss of vision, has been described (**Table 2**).

Table 2
Complications from pneumoperitoneum and Trendelenburg position during RALRP

Facial, eyelid, conjunctiva, tongue edema[42]
Corneal abrasion[42]
Conjunctival burns from reflux of stomach content[43]
Decreased visual field or blindness from posterior ischemic optical neuropathy[44]
Laryngeal edema requiring postoperative reintubation[45]
Pulmonary edema requiring postoperative reintubation[46]
Brachial plexus neuropathy[45]
Common peroneal, saphenous neuropathy[42]

Other considerations include limiting the amount of intravenous fluid to reduce facial edema and decrease urine output. The low intraoperative urine output maintains visualization during the vesicourethral anastomosis. We limit our first start patients to 1 L of saline solution until the anastomosis is completed, whereas later starts can receive 1.5 to 2 L because of increased dehydration before starting. Once the anastomosis is complete, the fluids are opened up until a total of 4 L is infused, which may be completed in the post-anesthesia care unit.

SURGICAL TECHNIQUE

There are many described technical variations of the RALRP that undergo constant modifications. A description of the various techniques is beyond the scope of this article; however, the major steps involved in a standard transperitoneal RALRP will be described. The goal of the surgery is to remove the entire cancer-containing prostate gland with the seminal vesicles and the ampulla of the vas while avoiding damages to other vital structures. Regardless of the approach, the RALRP proceeds in an anterograde fashion; the prostate is released from the bladder and the dissection proceeds "anterograde" in the direction of the laparoscope toward the urethra.

Port Placement

Before port placement, an 18-French Foley catheter is placed into the bladder on the sterile field. The port placement for a transperitoneal RALRP has evolved since the introduction of the updated S and SI robotic systems, which have smaller and less bulky patient side units. In general, pneumoperitoneum can be gained with a Veress needle or the Hasson technique. The camera port is placed at the level of the umbilicus. The left and right robotic arms are placed approximately 9 cm from the midline and 18 cm from the pubic symphysis. With the newer consoles, these measurements no longer need to be exact, and most surgeons use an approximate "hand width" to space the ports out properly. The fourth arm of the robot is usually placed just superior to the left anterior iliac spine and 9 cm from the left robotic arm. An assistant 12-mm port is also placed superior to the anterior iliac spine on the right side, and an additional 5-mm port is placed above and midway between the right robotic and camera port (**Fig. 2**). The table is maximally lowered, and the patient is placed in a steep Trendelenburg position.

Once the ports are placed, and attention is turned to docking the robot, it is important to drive and position the robot at an optimal distance and angle from the ports. This optimal distance is called the "sweet spot," and using the blue line and arrow on the camera arm can help judge how close to park the robot to the patient. Docking the robot is usually a coordinated effort between the patient-side assistant and the person driving the robot. Because the individual driving the robot often cannot see exactly where the robot needs to dock, it is the role of the scrubbed assistant to guide them in. Clear orientation as to which way to turn and how sharp to turn should be established before moving the robot. Consistent directions from the assistant and practice as the driver also aid in creating a smoother and easier docking experience. Once the robot is docked, the nursing team must make sure that the arms are not resting on the legs, feet, or other parts of the body. This is sometimes overlooked because of the surgical drapes.

Entering the space of Retzius

A 0° lens is initially used for the first part of the operation. A pair of monopolar scissors is used in the right hand, while a bipolar Maryland or PK is used as the left-handed

Port Placement of Robotic Radical Prostatectomies

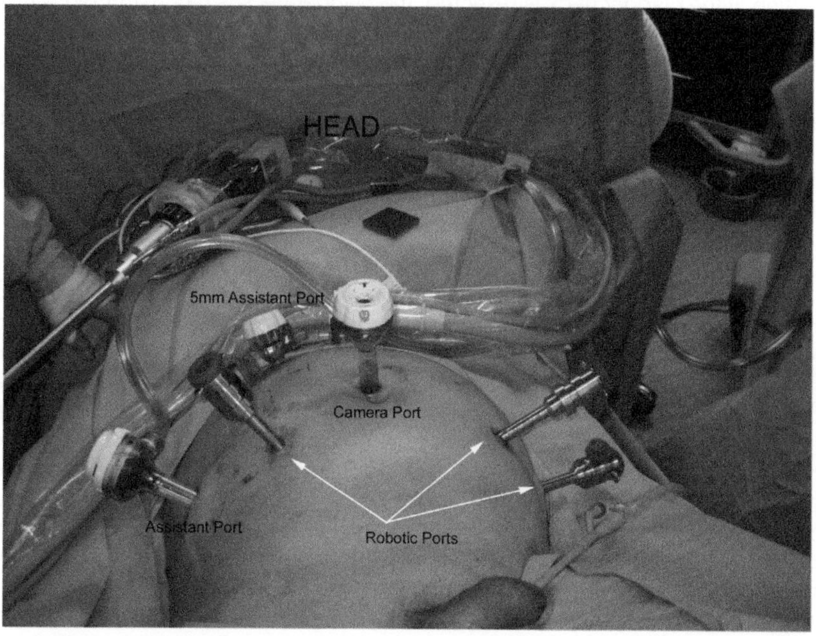

Fig. 2. Typical port placement for a RALRP. The camera port is placed 22 to 26 cm from the pubic symphsis at the level of the umbilicus. The remaining robotic ports are placed 9 cm lateral to the camera port. An additional 12-mm assistant port is placed just above the anterior superior iliac spine on the right side, and a 5-mm suction port is placed between the camera and right-sided robotic port in the upper abdomen.

instrument. A Prograsp forceps is often used for retraction in the fourth arm. If the surgeon decides to perform a posterior approach to dissecting the seminal vesicle and vas deferens, the patient's sigmoid colon is retracted out of the pelvis and the cul-de-sac is incised. With dissection, the vas deferens and the seminal vesicles are identified. The vas deferens on either side is divided, and the seminal vesicles are dissected off using Weck Hem- O- Lok Ligating Clips (Teleflex Medical, Research Triangle Park, NC, USA) to control the pedicles. Denonvilliers' fascia is then separated posteriorly off the prostate, releasing the attachments to the rectum. Attention is then turned anteriorly.

The peritoneum lateral to the medial umbilical ligament is taken down bilaterally to create a flap of the peritoneum including the bladder to enter the space of Retzius. The fat overlying the endopelvic fascia and the prostate is removed, and the endopelvic fascia on either side of the prostate is opened up sharply, and dissection is carried out to roll the prostate off the pelvic sidewall attachments. Once the dorsal venous complex has been adequately dissected out, a 1-0 polydioxanone (PDS) suture with a CT-1 needle is used to secure the dorsal venous complex. Alternatively, an endo-gastrointestinal anastomosis (GIA) vascular stapler may be used to staple and divide the dorsal venous complex instead of suturing.

Detaching the prostate from the bladder neck
Many surgeons change to a 30° down lens after securing the dorsal venous complex because it helps facilitate the visualization of the bladder-prostate junction. The

bladder neck is identified and incised, and attempts are made to preserve it during the dissection. If the bladder neck is resected, the bladder neck is reconstructed with 3-0 Vicryl sutures later. The Foley catheter is brought through the bladder neck, opening once the anterior dissection is completed, and the Foley is held up by the fourth arm of the robot along with gentle external Foley traction. The prostate is then completely detached from the bladder. The seminal vesicles and ampulla of the vas are then dissected out and grasped with the fourth arm and the prostate is retracted upward. Further dissection is carried out to free up residual prostate attachments to the rectum posteriorly.

Nerve sparing and division of prostate pedicles

Depending on the patient's clinical presentation, non-nerve–sparing, unilateral nerve-sparing, or bilateral nerve-sparing prostatectomies are performed. In the case of the non-nerve–sparing procedure, the prostate pedicles on either side are serially thinned out, clipped with Weck Hem- O- Lok Ligating Clips, and divided. A bipolar device such as the Enseal Trio Tissue Sealing Device, (Ethicon Endo- Surgery Inc, Cincinnati, OH, USA) or the robot bipolar instrument can be used to divide the prostate pedicles. In the case of a nerve-sparing procedure, the superficial fascia of the prostate is incised and separated from the prostate. This tissue is pushed down, and the prostate pedicles are then identified, clipped with Weck Hem- O- Lok Ligating Clips, and then divided, hugging the prostate. The attachments laterally are all taken[29] down eventually, sharply leaving the neurovascular bundle in place. The use of any thermo-electrical energy source of cutting and coagulating, or excess traction to the prostate or neurovascular bundle, is avoided because of potential injury to the neurovascular bundle.

Urethral division

After the prostate had been freed up on both sides and posteriorly, attention is then turned anteriorly. The dorsal venous complex is transected sharply. The urethra is identified. The apex of the prostate may be retracted back to expose a longer length of the urethra to preserve a good urethral length. The urethra is then transected sharply and the rectourethralis attachments are taken down to free up the entire prostate. The prostate is placed into the patient's right lower quadrant. Irrigation is carried out and inspection of the resection site is carried out. Any significant bleeding at this point may be controlled with 3-0 Vicryl suture ligature. If needed, the bladder neck is reconstructed with a 3-0 Vicryl suture.

Pelvic lymph node dissection

If pelvic lymph node dissection is indicated, attention is then turned to the patient's pelvic sidewall where the superficial fascia of the external iliac vein is incised sharply. This dissection is then carried down to identify the pelvic sidewall. All tissues between the external iliac vein and the obturator nerve are taken. The lymphatic channels going to the lymph node packet are clipped with Weck Hem- O- Lok Ligating Clips and divided sharply. A similar procedure is performed on both sides.

Vesicourethral anastomosis

Reapproximation of the rectourethralis, the cut layer of Denonvilliers' fascia, and the bladder (referred to as a Rocco stitch) is performed with a single "barbed" V-Lock 90 suture (Covidien, Mansfield, MA, USA). This method pulls the bladder neck closer to the urethral stump and may improve short-term incontinence. Once completed, the vesicourethral anastomosis is performed. A composite double-armed suture is made with two V-Lock 90 sutures. A running vesicourethral anastomosis is started posteriorly, which is carried anteriorly. A new 18-French Foley catheter is placed, and 10 mL is placed in the balloon. The bladder is irrigated to check for leakage and to clear the bladder of any blood clots. The catheter is then placed to gravity drainage.

Specimen retrieval and drain placement

The prostate is then placed in the specimen bag via the assistant's 12-mm port, and the string is eventually transferred to the 5-mm assistant port. There is no consensus on the use of an internal drain, which may help detect postoperative bleeding or urinary leak. If a drain is placed, the robotic fourth arm is undocked, and a 19-French Blake drain is placed through the fourth arm robot port and laid anterior to the bladder. All robotic instruments are removed at this point, and the robot is undocked. The umbilical incision is enlarged to allow specimen retrieval. The string from the 5-mm port is grasped through this incision with a finger and the specimen is extracted. The umbilical port site fascia is closed with a 0 Vicryl with a UR-6 needle. All other port sites are closed with subcuticular sutures. Local anesthesia is injected in each of the port sites, and each of the port sites is closed with Dermabond (Ethicon, Cincinnati, OH, USA). The drain is sutured in place using a nylon suture. At this point, the patient is awakened from anesthesia and taken to the recovery room.

POSTOPERATIVE CARE

After the procedure, the patient is monitored in the recovery room and eventually transferred to a hospital ward when criteria are met. In general, the patients are admitted for overnight observations. Typically the patient is administered intravenous ketorolac every 6 hours around the clock, and intravenous morphine or oral narcotics as needed for analgesia. The patient is kept on cefazolin until discharge. Although there is no clear consensus regarding antibiotic coverage postoperatively, patients are typically placed on ciprofloxacin 500 mg twice a day until the Foley catheter has been removed. The patient is given a clear liquid diet, which is advanced to a regular diet on postoperative day 1. An intraabdominal drain, if left in place, is removed on postoperative day 1 if there is no evidence of anastomotic urinary leak. The patient is educated on Foley catheter care and is discharged to home, usually on postoperative day 1, with leg bedside urinary drainage bags. On discharge, the patient is instructed to resume all preoperative medications except for anticoagulants, and is administered hydrocodone, docusate sodium, and ciprofloxacin.

After hospital discharge, the patient is seen for office follow-up in 10 to 14 days. A cystogram to assess for anastomotic leak can be considered, but it is not done routinely. The patients are asked to bring an adult diaper at the time of the follow-up. A physical examination is performed. The pathology report is reviewed with the patient. A voiding trial is performed by placing the patient on a toilet and filling up the bladder through the Foley catheter by gravity. The Foley catheter is removed when the patient reports sensation of urgency, and the patient is allowed to void. A bladder ultrasound is performed to check a post-void residual to ensure that the patient is able to empty his bladder. The patient is asked to resume the pelvic floor rehabilitation, and restart low-dose oral PDE-5 inhibitors twice a week. The patient is counseled again regarding the option of the use of the vacuum-assisted device and/or intracorporeal injection of vasoactive substance for erections. The patients are seen for follow-up again in 5 to 7 days. Subsequent follow-up involves monitoring patient's PSA levels starting 6 weeks after surgery, and the patient is seen every 3 months thereafter to continue to assess urinary and sexual functions. Typically, no further invasive intervention is recommended for urinary incontinence or erectile dysfunction for 1 or 2 years, respectively, after RALRP.

OUTCOME

Despite its popularity, there are questions on whether RALRP has real outcome advantages over RP, and whether these advantages justify the high cost of RALRP. The da Vinci surgical system may cost from US $1 million to $2.5 million for each unit.[30] There are also significant maintenance and disposable equipment costs.[30–32] Robotic surgery may be more time consuming than other surgical approaches. However, some of these costs may be offset by the potential decreased hospital stay and faster patient recovery.[31,32] Despite published reports of similar or superior oncologic, functional outcomes, complication rates, transfusion rates, and recovery when RALRP is compared with RRP, there are few randomized controlled trials to make a true determination.[33] The perceived benefits, partly due to aggressive marketing, even contribute to unrealistic patient expectations. In fact, it has been reported that patients who have undergone RALRP are 3 to 4 times as likely to be dissatisfied and regretful as patients undergoing RRP, even both groups had similar functional outcomes and side effects.[34]

Recent comparative studies between RALRP and RRP often show conflicting data (**Table 3**). This comparison is also difficult because there is a paucity of high-quality data from either surgical approach, no standardized data reporting is available, and most of the data come from centers highly specialized in prostate cancer treatment, which may not necessarily translate into a community setting. Although it is generally accepted that patients who underwent RALRP have less blood loss and faster functional recovery from the surgery, it appears that oncologic and functional outcome, regardless of approach, is highly dependent on surgeon training and experience. A RALRP performed by an expert surgeon has no significant health-related quality-of-life advantages over RRP also performed by an expert surgeon at 36 months after treatment.[35]

Despite the uncertainty over the superiority of the RALRP compared with other approaches, RALRP has revolutionized the method in which prostate cancer is treated. RALRP has become the most dominant surgical approach in the United States, with a vast majority of all radical prostatectomies being performed using the da Vinci system. As evident by the exponential growth in the number of robotic systems available, and literature concerning the use of the robot for the prostate, urologic surgeons have clearly accepted and continue to promote the RALRP as first therapy for prostate cancer.

ROBOT-ASSISTED LAPAROSCOPIC RENAL SURGERY

With the advent and rise in popularity of the da Vinci surgical system for the treatment of prostate cancer, the application of robot-assisted laparoscopic renal surgery was quickly realized. The robot afforded even open surgeons the ability to operate laparoscopically and significantly reduced the learning curve for some laparo-scopic procedures.[36] Its application to laparoscopic radical nephrectomy, how-ever, has been limited because of the cost effectiveness of standard laparoscopy over a robot-assisted approach and the established familiarity and ease of a laparoscopic approach for a procedure that is completely extirpative and thus requires no suturing.

Laparoscopic partial nephrectomy and pyeloplasty, on the other hand, has enjoyed a significant increase in adoption via the da Vinci surgical system largely because of

Table 3

Recent comparative studies comparing outcome data from different prostatectomy approaches

Author and Year	Conclusion
Lowrance et al (2010)[47]	RALRP and RRP have similar postoperative morbidity and mortality. LRP with or without robot assistance has shorter length of stay and lower risk of bladder neck or urethral obstruction.
Coelho et al (2010)[48]	RRP, LRP, RALRP have similar complication rates. LRP and RALRP have decreased blood loss, transfusion rate, and PSM rates. RALRP has lower PSM rates and higher continence rates compared with RRP and LRP.
Williams et al (2010)[50]	Nerve-sparing RALRP has higher PSM rates compared with nerve-sparing RRP, but non- nerve–sparing RALRP has lower PSM rates compared with non-nerve–sparing RRP.
Malcolm et al (2010)[37]	RALRP has no significant health-related quality-of-life advantages over RRP.
Barocas et al (2010)[17]	RALRP and RRP have similar biochemical recurrence rates.
Ficarra et al (2009)[49]	RALRP had lower transfusion rate, shorter urethral catheterization, length of stay, fewer perioperative complications but longer operative times. PSM rates are similar between RALRP and RRP.
Berryhill et al (2008)[19]	Compared with RP, RALRP had lower blood loss and transfusion rates, shorter urethral catheter time, less PSM, and a lower complication rate. Continence rate appeared to be better at 3 and 6 months between RALRP and RRP. Potency and operative times are similar.
Miller et al (2007)[18]	Patient who underwent RALRP had less intraoperative blood loss, had better physical well-being postoperatively, and more rapid return to baseline compared with RRP.

Abbreviations: LRP, laparoscopic radical prostatectomy; PSM, positive surgical margin; RALRP, robot assisted laparoscopic radical prostatectomy; RRP, retropubic prostatectomy.

its reconstructive nature. The robot offers a number of different tools that can allow for precise tumor excision and complex renal reconstruction. Since its introduction in 2004,[37] a growing number of institutions have demonstrated success with robot-assisted laparoscopic partial nephrectomy, reporting equivalent or improved perioperative outcomes in comparison with laparoscopic partial nephrectomy.[3,38] Advantages offered by the da Vinci platform such as 7 degrees of freedom, 3D vision, and tremor filtration have furthermore shortened the learning curve for partial nephrectomy. These advantages have also contributed to establishing the robotic approach as the "gold standard" for upper tract urinary reconstruction, such as pyeloplasty.[12,39]

Robotic renal surgery is not nearly as common as RALRP, but has some unique peri-operative features that require some examination. Unlike prostate surgery, vascular complications during renal surgery can be catastrophic. Currently the robot can be used for nephron-sparing surgery, radical nephrectomy, pyeloplasty, and various other extirpative or reconstructive procedures. Unlike the prostate section above, we will not focus on a specific disease entity while examining the use of the robot for renal surgery. Instead, the general principles involved with all robotic renal surgery will be examined.

Patient Positioning for Robotic Renal Surgery

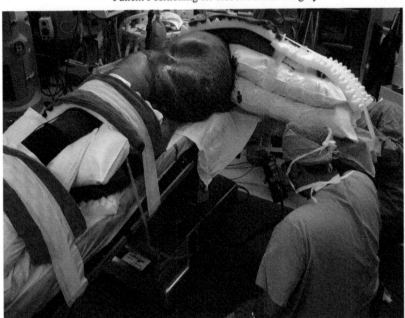

Fig. 3. Lateral decubitis positioning typical for robotic renal surgery.

Patient Positioning and Preparation

Patient position is essential for robotic renal surgery. Improper positioning can lead to neuropraxias or rhabdomyolysis. It can also limit the functionality of the robot by creating problems with docking the robot, and using the robotic instruments. For most robotic renal surgeries, the patient is positioned in a 45° modified lateral decubitis position or in the full flank position for traditional transperitoneal access. If the surgery is to be performed through the retroperitoneal space, the patient is placed in the full flank position. An axillary roll must be placed, and extra padding is used at the hip, knee, and foot, as well as the arms, which are supported on an arm board **(Fig. 3)**. The table is slightly flexed and the patient is secured firmly to the bed with foam and heavy taping at the greater trochanter of the hip, the calf, and over the upside of the shoulder. The kidney rest is not activated or used during the procedure. An orogastric tube should be placed and kept on low, intermittent suction throughout the case, and a Foley catheter should be inserted before positioning.

Transperitoneal surgery

Port placement for most transperitoneal robotic renal surgeries generally follows the same pattern; however, unlike RALRP, there is often less working space and decreased functionality of the robot if the ports are not positioned properly. After positioning the patient, we generally insufflate the abdomen with either a Veress needle or via the Hasson technique. We then mark out anatomic landmarks after insufflation, because these points often shift during insufflation. As seen in **Fig. 4**, the midline, the paramedian line (just lateral to the rectus muscle), costal margin, and pelvic outline are all marked out. For most transperitoneal surgery, the camera is

Port Placement for a Standard Transperitoneal Robotic Renal Surgery

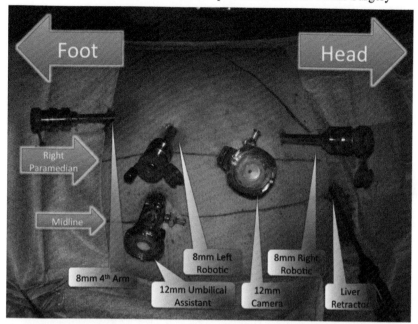

Fig. 4. Typical port placement for robotic renal surgery (all types). On the right side a liver retractor is needed as seen above.

placed at the paramedian line approximately 6 cm above the umbilicus. The left and right robotic arms are then placed 8 cm away. A fourth arm is usually placed just off the anterior superior iliac spine and finally the assistant port is hidden in the umbilicus. For a right-sided surgery, a small 5-mm port can be used to retract the liver as seen in the image. All ports are placed under direct vision.

For a standard transperitoneal surgery, the robot is usually moved into position at an angle over the patient's shoulder. This often requires the operating room table to be unlocked and the bed adjusted to accommodate the robot. Once the robot is docked, the abdomen is inspected and access to the retroperitoneum is gained after taking down the white line of Toldt. This maneuver allows the colon and its mesentery to be medially reflected and gains access directly onto Gerota's fascia. Once Gerota's fascia is properly identified, the attachments to the colon and mesentery of the colon can be reflected medially to reveal the great vessels and ureter. At this point the operation can continue as needed depending on the surgery type.

Retroperitoneal surgery
Retroperitoneal surgery, especially when using the robotic system, presents a large number of difficulties. The retroperitoneal space is very small with a very limited working space. Because of the small working space, there is often a large number of instrument clashing, and the assistant has very little room to stay comfortable and work. However, the retroperitoneal approach is ideal for posterior located renal tumors when performing a partial nephrectomy; it avoids the peritoneal cavity in the patient with multiple previous surgeries or other contraindications to transperitoeneal surgery; and it is associated with quicker recovery and less postoperative pain.

Port Placement for a Retroperitoneal Robotic Renal Surgery

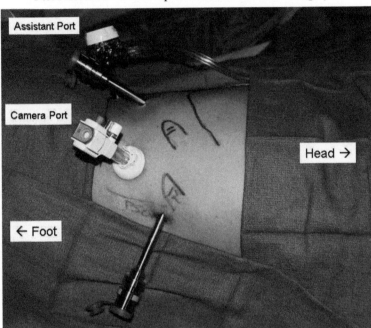

Fig. 5. Typical port placement for retroperitoneal robotic surgery.

With the patient in the full flank position, access to the retroperitoneum is gained with an incision just under the tip of the 12th rib. The muscle and facial layers are dissected down until the retroperitoneal fat is encountered. Using blunt finger dissection, a space is developed over the psoas muscle. A balloon dilator is then used to create a working space, and the remaining ports are placed under direct visual guidance, as seen in **Fig. 5**. The right and left robotic arms are placed about 8 cm off of the camera. One port is at the costovertebral angle, just above the psoas muscle. The medial arm often requires some dissection of the peritoneum to create enough space to place the port without entering the peritoneal cavity. An assistant port is placed inferior medially and usually just above the hip.

When performing a surgery through the retroperitoneal approach, the robot is docked directly over the patient's head. The anesthesia team must be cognizant of the issues of access to the endotracheal tube, once the robot is in position; however, there is usually ample room to access the tube underneath the robotic arms. Overall, proper port placement and docking are required to use the enhanced features of the robotic system without limiting its functionality because of external clashing or limit the robotic arms because of improper positioning.

Postoperative care

With all robotic renal surgery, the orogastric tube is removed before extubation. When the patient is fully awake, clear liquids are provided and the diet is advanced as tolerated. Sequential intermittent compression stockings remain in place until the patient is ambulating. The Foley catheter can be removed on the first postoperative day depending on the type of surgery. Complete blood count and serum electrolytes are checked immediately postoperatively and on the morning of postoperative day 1. In general, patients are discharged on the evening of postoperative day 1 or the morning of postoperative day 2 for standard renal surgery.

Management of intraoperative complications

The full intraoperative complications associated with any laparoscopic or robotic renal procedure are beyond the scope of this article; however, the most concerning will be mentioned. Cardiac arrest is extremely rare and usually associated with a vaso-vagal reaction after insufflating the abdomen. It is not specific to renal surgery and can best be treated by desufflating the abdomen.[40,41] An air embolism, which is usually the result of improperly placing a Veress needle or trocar into a major vein, is also extremely unusual; however, if suspected, the right flank should be placed up.

Vascular injuries are a major concern, especially during robotic renal surgery. Because there are great vessels surrounding the kidney, careful dissection and good preoperative planning by examining the CT or MRI imaging before the procedure are essential to avoiding major vascular injuries. Venous bleeding can be initially managed with increasing the intraabdominal pressure to 20 to 25 mm Hg. This is usually sufficient to decrease the extent of the bleed. The injury should then be tamponaded with a suction device or Kittner sponge. A robotic bowel grasper or fenestrated bipolar can also be used to grasp the area of bleeding, which will allow time for the team to prepare for the repair. The robot enables the surgeon precise movements and can easily be used to repair major vascular injuries with fine suture, but it requires a deft assistant and support from the perioperative nursing staff. In the face of arterial bleeding, increasing the pressure is of no help. One has to quickly tamponade the area of arterial bleeding. If that is not successful, then a conversion to an open procedure is immediately indicated. The perioperative nursing team must be capable of quickly moving the robot out in the event of an emergent conversion to open surgery.

Bowel injury is most commonly due to electrosurgical injury, especially when the colon is reflected during transperitoneal renal surgery. Making sure the protecting sheathing is not violated on the robotic monopolar scissors can limit the chance of these unnecessary injuries from occurring. If recognized intraoperatively, the injured area needs to be widely excised and a suture repair is done, which can be performed robotically. On the right side, the duodenum is at significant risk for injury. It is recommended that if there is an injury to the duodenum, a patch of omentum should be used over the repair and a drain should be left in place. In either case, intraoperative consultation with a general surgeon is recommended. A case time of more than 4 hours along with deficient padding, improper positioning, or use of the kidney rest can lead to neuropraxias or rhabdomyolysis.[40,41] Any suspected nerve injury should be investigated immediately by the anesthesia team as well as by neurology. Procedures lasting more than 5 hours, especially in the obese male patient, risk the development of rhabdomyolysis. A key symptom that this is occurring is when the patient, upon awakening, complains of significant discomfort over the contralateral hip.

Postoperative complications

Postoperative hemorrhage can occur after any robotic renal surgery. It is characterized by a greater than 10 point drop in hematocrit in the postoperative labs and warrants immediate exploration. Acute hemorrhage is invariably due to an arterial bleed. For patients with a gradual drop in hematocrit during the first couple of postoperative days, exploration should be considered. However, this is usually due to venous bleeding, and a specific point of bleeding is commonly not identified.[40]

A delayed bowel injury should be considered if there is increasing abdominal discomfort or low-grade fever. The bowel sounds may be normal on physical examination. Of note, a normal or low white blood count with a left shift may be a harbinger of a bowel injury. A CT scan with oral contrast with immediate and delayed films in 4 hours should be obtained to rule out a bowel injury. Treatment when the injury is discovered in the immediate postoperative period is to reestablish the laparoscopic ports and repair the injury laparoscopically or robotically. Delayed bowel injury that can take upwards of 17 days postoperatively to present will often require open exploration to identify the site of injury and repair it.

SUMMARY

The da Vinci robotic system has revolutionized urology and created a paradigm shift in the management of prostate cancer and most other urologic diseases. Its explosive growth in the field of urology is a product of the ease of use and ability to enable even open surgeons, with limited laparoscopic skills, the ability to provide minimally invasive surgery to their patients. Although there are some drawbacks to the system, such as the high costs to purchase and maintain, the robot will certainly be an integral part of urology in the future.

ACKNOWLEDGMENTS

We thank the Queen's Medical Center internal OR. Data are courtesy of Maggie Magee, RN. The port placement photos are courtesy of Daniel Eun, MD.

REFERENCES

1. Annual Report 2009. Intutive Surgical.
2. Brandina R, Gill IS. Robotic partial nephrectomy: new beginnings. Eur Urol 2010;57: 778–9.
3. Benway BM, Bhayani SB. Robot-assisted partial nephrectomy: evolution and recent advances. Curr Opin Urol 2010;20:119–24.
4. Pruthi RS, Wallen EM. Current status of robotic prostatectomy: promises fulfilled. J Urol 2009;181:2420–1.
5. Vira MA, Richstone L. Robotic cystectomy: its time has come. J Urol 2010;183: 421–2.
6. Richards KA, Kader AK, Hemal AK. Robotic radical cystectomy: where are we today, where will we be tomorrow? Sci World J 2010;10:2215–7.
7. Mansour AM, Marshall SJ, Arnone ED, et al. Status of robot-assisted radical cystectomy. Can J Urol 2010;17:5002–11.
8. McDougall EM, Clayman RV, Elashry OM. Laparoscopic radical nephrectomy for renal tumor: The Washington University experience. J Urol 1996;155:1180–5.
9. Kerbl K, Clayman RV, McDougall EM, et al. Transperitoneal nephrectomy for benign disease of the kidney—a comparison of laparoscopic and open surgical techniques. Urology 1994;43:607–13.
10. Wexner SD, Bergamaschi R, Lacy A, et al. The current status of robotic pelvic surgery: results of a multinational interdisciplinary consensus conference. Surg Endosc 2009; 23:438–43.
11. Moorthy K, Munz Y, Dosis A, et al. Dexterity enhancement with robotic surgery. Surg Endosc 2004;18:790–5.
12. Mehta S, Dasgupta P, Challacombe BJ. Robotic reconstructive urology: possibilities for the urological surgeon beyond the prostate. BJU Int 2010;106:1247–8.

13. Ahlering TE, Skarecky D, Lee D, et al. Successful transfer of open surgical skills to a laparoscopic environment using a robotic interface: initial experience with laparoscopic radical prostatectomies. J Urol 2003;170:1738–41.

14. Gautam G, Shalhav AL. Robotic prostatectomy: not just marketing hype and here to stay. J Urol 2010;183:859–61.

15. Andriole GL, Grubb RL, Buys SS, et al. Mortality results from a randomized prostate-cancer screening trial. N Engl J Med 2009;360:1310.

16. Schroeder FH, Hugosson J, Roobol MJ, et al. Screening and prostate-cancer mortality in a randomized European study. N Engl J Med 2009;360:1320–8.

17. Barocas DA, Salem S, Kordan Y, et al. Robotic assisted laparoscopic prostatectomies versus radical retropubic prostatectomies for clinically localized prostate cancer: comparison of short-term biochemical recurrence-free survival. J Urol 2010;183:990–6.

18. Miller J, Smith A, Kouba E, et al. Prospective evaluation of short-term impact and recovery of health related quality of life in men undergoing robotic assisted laparoscopic radical prostatectomies versus open radical prostatectomies. J Urol 2007;178:854–8.

19. Berryhill R, Jhaveri J, Yadav R, et al. Robotic prostatectomy: a review of outcomes compared with laparoscopic and open approaches. Urology 2008;72:15–23.

20. Orvieto MA, Coelho RF, Chauhan S, et al. Erectile dysfunction after robot-assisted radical prostatectomies. Expert Rev Anticancer Ther 2010;10:747–54.

21. Montorsi F, McCullough A. Efficacy of sildenafil citrate in men with erectile dysfunction following radical prostatectomies: a systematic review of clinical data. J Sex Med 2005;2:658–67.

22. McCullough AR, Hellstrom WG, Wang R, et al. Recovery of erectile function after nerve sparing radical prostatectomies and penile rehabilitation with nightly intraurethral alprostadil versus sildenafil citrate. J Urol 2010;183:2451–6.

23. Awad H, Santilli S, Ohr M, et al. The effects of steep Trendelenburg positioning on intraocular pressure during robotic radical prostatectomies. Anesth Analg 2009;109:473–8.

24. Hewer CL. The physiology and complications of the Tendelenburg position. Can Med Assoc J 1956;74:285–8.

25. El-Galley R, Hammontree L, Urban D, et al. Anesthesia for laparoscopic donor nephrectomy: is nitrous oxide contraindicated? J Urol 2007;178:225–7.

26. Kalmar AF, Foubert L, Hendrickx JFA, et al. Influence of steep Trendelenburg position and CO_2 pneumoperitoneum on cardiovascular, cerebrovascular, and respiratory homeostasis during RALRP. Br J Anaesth 2010;104:433–9.

27. Irvine M, Patil V. Anaesthesia for robot-assisted laparoscopic surgery. Cont Edu Anaesth Crit Care & Pain 2009;9:125–9.

28. Gainsburg DM, Wax D, Reich DL, et al. Intraoperative management of robotic-assisted versus open radical prostatectomies. JSLS 2010;14:1–5.

29. Gautam G, Rocco B, Patel VR, et al. Posterior rhabdosphincter reconstruction during robot-assisted radical prostatectomy: critical analysis of techniques and outcomes. Urology 2010;73:734–41.

30. Smith A, Kurpad R, Lal A, et al. Cost analysis of robotic versus open radical cystectomy for bladder cancer. J Urol 2010;183:505–9.

31. Barbash GI, Glied SA. New technology and health care costs—the case of robot-assisted surgery. N Engl J Med 2010;363:701–4.

32. Bolenz C, Gupta A, Hotze T, et al. Cost comparison of robotic, laparoscopic, and open radical prostatectomies for prostate cancer. Eur Urol 2010;57:453–8.

33. Kang DC, Hardee MJ, Fesperman SF, et al. Low quality of evidence for robot-assisted laparoscopic prostatectomies: results of a systematic review of the published literature. Eur Urol 2010;57:930–7.

34. Schroeck FR, Krupski TL, Sun L, et al. Satisfaction and regret after open retropubic or robot-assisted laparoscopic radical prostatectomies. Eur Urol 2008;54:785–93.

35. Malcolm JB, Fabrizio MD, Barone BB, et al. Quality of life after open or RALRP, cryoablation or brachytherapy for localized prostate cancer. J Urol 2010;183:1822–8.

36. Zorn KC, Orvieto MA, Gong EM, et al. Robotic radical prostatectomy learning curve of a fellowship-trained laparoscopic surgeon. J Endourol 2007;21:441–7.

37. Gettman MT, Blute ML, Chow GK, et al. Robotic-assisted laparoscopic partial nephrectomy: technique and initial clinical experience with daVinci robotic system. Urology 2004;64:914–8.

38. Benway BM, Bhayani SB, Rogers CG, et al. Robot assisted partial nephrectomy versus laparoscopic partial nephrectomy for renal tumors: a multi-institutional analysis of perioperative outcomes. J Urol 2009;182:866–72.

39. Braga LHP, Pace K, DeMaria J, et al. Systematic review and meta-analysis of robotic-assisted versus conventional laparoscopic pyeloplasty for patients with ureteropelvic junction obstruction: effect on operative time, length of hospital stay, postoperative complications, and success rate. Eur Urol 2009;56:848–57.

40. Capelouto CC, Kavoussi LR. Complications of laparoscopic surgery. Urology 1993; 42:2–12.

41. Vallancien G, Cathelineau X, Baumert H, et al. Complications of transperitoneal laparoscopic surgery in urology: review of 1,311 procedures at a single center. J Urol 2002;168:23–6.

42. Costello TG, Webb P. Anaesthesia for robot-assisted anatomic prostatectomy. Experience at a single institution. Anaesth Intensive Care 2006;34:787–92.

43. Conacher ID, Soomro NA, Rix D. Anaesthesia for laparoscopic urological surgery. Br J Anaesth 2004;93:859–64.

44. Weber ED, Colyer MH, Lesser RL, Subramanian PR. Posterior ischemic optic neuropathy after minimally invasive prostatectomy. J Neuroophthalmol 2007;27:282–7.

45. Phong SVN, Koh LKD. Anaesthesia for robotic-assisted radical prostatectomy: considerations for laparoscopy in the Trendelenburg postion. Anaesth Intensive Care 2007;35:281–5.

46. Hong JY, Oh YJ, Rha KH, et al. Pulmonary edema after da Vinci-assisted laparoscopic radical prostatectomy: a case report. J Clin Anesth 2010;22:370–2.

47. Lowrance WT, Elkin EB, Jacks LM, et al. Comparative effectiveness of prostate cancer surgical treatments: a population based analysis of postoperative outcomes. J Urol 2010;183:1366–72.

48. Coelho RF, Rocco B, Patel MB, et al. Retropubic, laparoscopic, and robot-assisted radical prostatectomy: a critical review of outcomes reported by high-volume center. J Endourol 2010;24:2003–15.

49. Ficarra V, Novara G, Artibani W, et al. Retropubic laparoscopic, and robot-assisted radical prostatectomy: a systemic review and cumulative analysis of comparative studies. Eur Urol 2009;55:1037–63.

50. Williams SB, Chen MH, D'Amico AV, et al. Radical retropubic prostectomy and robot-assisted laparoscopic prostatectomy: likelihood of positive surgical margin(s). J Urol 2009;76:1097–101.

Robotic Liver Surgery

Kamran Idrees, MD, David L. Bartlett, MD*

KEYWORDS
- Robotic • Liver • Resection • Hepaticojejunostomy
- Surgery

The introduction of minimally invasive techniques has dramatically transformed surgery in the past 2 decades. This approach is shown to be beneficial in reducing the length of hospital stay, improving cosmetic results, and decreasing postoperative pain in all the surgical specialties compared with conventional open operations.[1–3] These advanced minimally invasive procedures require surgeons to have highly developed laparoscopic skills, including suturing, knot tying, and complex bimanual manipulation. However, conventional laparoscopic surgery has its own limitations, including reduced freedom of movement within the abdominal cavity and 2-dimensional view of a 3-dimensional operative field. In addition, the laparoscopic instruments provide surgeons with reduced precision and poor ergonomics.[4–6] These limitations translate into a significant learning curve, requiring a lot of time and effort to develop and maintain such advanced laparoscopic skills.[6,7] These shortcomings of laparoscopic surgery were the impetus behind the development of robotic surgery.

Robotic surgery allows surgeons to perform advanced laparoscopic procedures with greater ease. Similar to a human hand, the robotic articulating laparoscopic instruments translate the natural movements of the surgeon's hand into precise movements inside the abdominal cavity. The 3-dimensional view of the operative field along with 7° of freedom and tremor filtration allows the surgeon with wristlike dexterity to perform delicate dissection and precise intracorporeal suturing. These significant advantages of robotic surgery have expanded the scope of surgical procedures that can be performed through minimally invasive techniques.

Liver surgery was nonexistent in the beginning of the twentieth century because of the high propensity for bleeding and inherent friability of the liver. The improved understanding of liver anatomy and knowledge of its regenerative capability set the stage for the development of liver surgery in the middle of the twentieth century. Subsequent advancements in anesthesia, critical care, transfusion medicine, postoperative care, and enhanced diagnostic imaging by computed tomography and magnetic resonance imaging scans have transformed liver surgery to be performed routinely with reduced morbidity and mortality by the end of the last century. The

A version of this article was previously published in *Surgical Clinics* 90:4.
Division of Surgical Oncology, Department of Surgery, University of Pittsburgh Medical Center Cancer Pavilion, 5150 Centre Avenue, Suite 414, Pittsburgh, PA, USA
* Corresponding author.
E-mail address: bartdl@upmc.edu

technological advancements in the liver parenchymal transection techniques with the help of precoagulating devices, ultrasonic aspiration dissector, improved surface coagulators along with improved patient selection, and radiographic staging have paved the way for laparoscopic liver surgery. Laparoscopic liver surgery is increasingly being performed over the past several years, although it was more slowly embraced than the minimally invasive surgery revolution in gastrointestinal surgery.[8–13] Laparoscopic liver surgery offers the same universal benefits of minimally invasive surgery, such as better cosmesis, reduced duration of hospitalization, and less postoperative pain.[14–16] The technique has been shown to be as safe and feasible in experienced hands. However, the restrictive movement of laparoscopic instruments, limited by fixed pivot point with only 4° of freedom and 2-dimensional view, limits its utility in hepatobiliary surgery with a complex repertoire of operations. Robotic surgery was developed to address some of these inherent limitations of laparoscopic surgery and in this article the authors' preview the potential scope of robotics in hepatobiliary surgery.

ADVANTAGES AND DISADVANTAGES OF ROBOTIC SURGERY

The da Vinci Surgical System (Intuitive Surgical, Inc, Sunnyvale, CA, USA) is the only commercially available therapeutic robotic system in the market, which was approved by the US Food and Drug Administration for use in surgery. The system is being used in various surgical subspecialties, including urology, gynecology, and colorectal and cardiothoracic surgery. The robotic surgical platform has several pros and cons (**Table 1**). The system provides more fluid movement because of tremor filtration, scaling of the movements, and articulating instruments with 7° of freedom, which results in increased dexterity to perform delicate dissection and precise intracorporeal suturing. This additional dexterity provided by wristed instruments is also of paramount importance in complex surgical procedures in difficult anatomic locations (**Fig. 1**). The 3-dimensional stereoscopic view with adjustable magnification provides superior visualization compared with standard laparoscopy and open surgery. The camera is on a stable camera platform and directly controlled by the surgeon, eliminating the need for an assistant to hold the video camera. The comfortable seated operating posture reduces fatigue and physical stress on the surgeon as compared with conventional laparoscopy, which often requires the surgeon to assume unnatural postures (**Fig. 2**). The coaxial alignment of eyes, hands, and tool tip images along with intuitive translation of the instrument handle to the tip movement not only eliminates mirror-image effect but also improves hand-eye coordination. The surgical robots are, however, not without their own disadvantages. These systems are costly; are bulky, requiring a lot of operating room space and an inefficient switch of instruments; have limited trocar placement options, making it difficult to switch

Table 1	
Pros and cons of robotic surgery	
Pros	**Cons**
• Advanced technology	• Expense
• Complex movements	• Learning curve
• Improved visibility	• Increased duration of case
• Better camera control	• Lack of tactile feedback
• Enhanced suturing capability	• Need for skilled assistant
• Future improvements in technology	• Difficult conversion to open

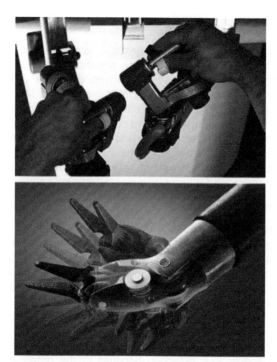

Fig. 1. The hand controls for the da Vinci system and the degrees of movement of the robotic instruments are demonstrated here. (*Courtesy of* Intuitive Surgical, Inc, Sunnyvale, CA, USA; with permission.)

operative fields during a procedure; and most importantly lack tactile feedback.[17–19] Acquisition and annual maintenance of these surgical robots is an expensive proposition. Operating times are greatly increased if the operative field is switched during the procedure, requiring patient repositioning, moving, and redocking of the

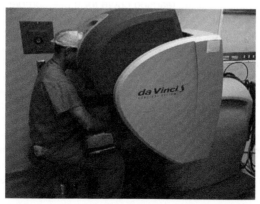

Fig. 2. The primary surgeon sits comfortably at the console while performing the robotic surgery.

robot. The absence of tactile feedback can result in tissue injury as well as breaking of suture.

Many surgeons attempt to assess or question the advantages of robotic surgery over straight laparoscopic surgery. Although patient outcome is improved with a minimally invasive approach, the use of a robot does not provide incremental improvement over straight laparoscopy for most procedures. Many skilled laparoscopists can perform complex suturing and complex procedures without the aid of the robot. However, the lesson learned from the prostate experience is that the use of a robot leads to an easier and faster sutured urethral anastomosis and more surgeons can perform this anastomosis safer and faster robotically than with straight laparoscopy.[20,21] The robot should be looked at as a new advanced tool to improve the minimally invasive approach for complex procedures such as liver resections.

ROBOTIC LIVER RESECTION

Technological advancement and improvement in laparoscopy have resulted in exponential increase in the number of laparoscopic liver resections across the world in the past few years.[8-13] Improved cosmetic results, shorter hospitalization, and less postoperative pain are compelling reasons to perform minimally invasive liver resection, especially for benign hepatic lesions. An international consensus conference was convened to evaluate the status of laparoscopic liver surgery.[22] According to this consensus report, the best indications for laparoscopic liver resection were solitary lesions, 5 cm or less, located in the peripheral liver segments (segments 2–6), whereas lesions adjacent to major vessels or near the liver hilum were not considered suitable for laparoscopic liver resection because of the potential risk of massive bleeding and the potential need for biliary reconstruction. Malignant tumors (colorectal liver metastases and hepatocellular carcinoma [HCC]) are not a contraindication to minimally invasive resection as demonstrated in various comparative studies, as long as there is no compromise in the oncologic integrity of the procedure. Although robotic liver surgery was not discussed in the consensus conference manuscript, the same rules can be applied to the technique as long as patient safety and oncologic results are not compromised.

Robotic liver surgery will broaden the scope of minimally invasive liver surgery by overcoming some of the limitations of conventional laparoscopy, including the difficulty to suture bleeding hepatic parenchyma laparoscopically, to perform complex hilar dissections, and to perform liver resections requiring biliary-enteric reconstructions, and by minimizing the learning curve for these complex procedures. One of the major concerns of laparoscopic liver resection is major bleeding from vascular structures within the parenchyma. This fear of uncontrolled bleeding has deterred liver surgeons from performing major liver resections using a minimally invasive technique. Several features of the da Vinci robot are extremely useful in controlling and definitely managing bleeding without conversion to an open surgery. These features include the use of 3 robotic arms by the same operating surgeon with use of articulating instruments to be locked in place as vascular clamps with the ability to perform intracorporeal suturing and tying in difficult locations. The capability of locking the articulating instruments in place as a substitute for vascular clamp is invaluable because it gives the anesthesia team time to resuscitate the patient and the surgical team to formulate a plan to manage the situation. The da Vinci surgical robot was used to repair a large vena caval tear after a staple misfire during a robot-assisted liver resection.[23]

With an increase in the incidence of HCC as a result of hepatitis C and the nonalcoholic steatohepatitis epidemic, more patients will benefit from minimally invasive surgical resection because of limited availability of liver allografts.[22] Minimally invasive liver surgery, which results in less postoperative adhesions making subsequent dissection relatively easy, is especially useful in patients with HCC who may require repetitive surgery or future transplantation. Two case series have shown the feasibility of robot-assisted left lateral hepatic segmentectomies.[24,25] As surgeons' experience with robotics improves, major hepatectomies will be more commonplace at busy liver centers. The delicate dissection that can be performed with the robotic platform to achieve inflow and outflow control and safe parenchymal transection will be recognized as a distinct advantage over laparoscopic instruments for major liver resections. Although robotic liver surgery is in its infancy, the advantages offered by surgical robots will undoubtedly expand its use for this purpose in the future.

ROBOTIC BILIARY-ENTERIC RECONSTRUCTION

The precision, steadiness, and manual dexterity conferred by robotic surgery make it ideal for biliary dissection and biliary-enteric anastomosis. Hence, the technique can be used for a multitude of benign conditions including choledochal cyst excision, benign common bile duct strictures, and biliary atresia.[26–28] One can not only perform fine dissection within the portal triad but also carry out intricate suturing required for the Roux-en-Y bilioenteric anastomosis. The anastomosis has to be performed meticulously so as to not compromise the anastomotic integrity and to avoid any technical errors that result in anastomotic stricture formation from improper suturing or vascular compromise. Several case reports and series have been published reporting the safety and feasibility of robotic biliary surgery in adults as well as in pediatric population for choledochal cyst disease and biliary atresia. Successful accomplishment of cyst excision along with biliary-enteric anastomosis and Kasai portoenterostomy has been reported in these studies.[26–28] Despite the fact that the first laparoscopic choledochal cyst excision with Roux-en-Y hepaticojejunostomy was performed in 1995, these procedures are still not routinely performed, which is an attestation to the fact that although these complex biliary procedures can be performed with conventional laparoscopic technique they are extremely difficult and challenging.[29] This disadvantage is secondary to the restrictive movement of laparoscopic instruments, combined with the fulcrum effect of laparoscopy, poor ergonomics, and compromised dexterity.

Robotic surgery overcomes all these shortcomings of conventional laparoscopy. Another advantage of performing these procedures through a minimally invasive technique as opposed to an open surgery is less postoperative adhesions, making subsequent surgery such as liver transplantation after failed Kasai procedure possibly easier. Robotic surgery does have its own set of disadvantages as discussed earlier, including the lack of tactile sensation, which makes it difficult for the surgeon to gauge the tension while manipulating and maneuvering tissue or suture.

COMBINED ROBOT-ASSISTED LIVER AND COLORECTAL RESECTION

Liver metastases are diagnosed simultaneously in 15% to 20% of newly diagnosed colorectal cancers.[30–32] Simultaneous colorectal and liver resection is performed at specialized institutes with low morbidity and mortality in carefully selected patients. This approach has shown to be advantageous in terms of oncologic outcomes, quality of life, as well as cost-effectiveness.[33,34] Laparoscopic colorectal surgery is being increasingly performed ever since adequacy of oncologic resections has been found to be similar in several large prospective randomized trials.[35,36] Based on comparable oncologic results and added advantages of improved visualization, enhanced dexterity, and great ergonomics, robotic surgery is being used more often in colorectal cancer, especially in rectal surgery. Wristed articulating instruments with a 3-dimensional view along with 7° of freedom provides increased maneuverability in anatomically challenging locations such as a narrow male pelvis and infradiaphragmatic hepatic vein isolation. Another benefit of robotic surgery is the ability to accurately suture intracorporeally to ligate bleeding vessels or to reinforce staple line in the pelvis. This minimally invasive approach has the potential advantage of improved early outcome after a major operation and thus allows for early administration of adjuvant chemotherapy. A pilot study has been performed demonstrating the safety and feasibility of robot-assisted simultaneous liver and colorectal resection.[37]

ROBOTIC HEPATIC ARTERY INFUSION PUMP PLACEMENT

Liver is the most common site of metastasis for colorectal cancer, and 60% of patients with colorectal cancer eventually develop hepatic metastases.[30,31] Together, HCC and intrahepatic cholangiocarcinoma account for most primary liver cancers.[38,39] Surgical resection is the most effective therapy for colorectal liver metastases as well as primary liver cancers; however, only a subset of patients are candidates for curative resection. Unlike systemic chemotherapy for colorectal metastases, the results of systemic therapy for primary liver cancers are disappointing.[40–42] Liver-directed therapy with the help of a surgically implanted hepatic arterial infusion pump provides an attractive option because it is not limited by tumor size, location, multifocality, or proximity to vascular structures, and higher doses can be given with little systemic side effects.[43] Hepatic artery infusion (HAI) therapy has been shown to be effective and safe for unresectable, isolated colorectal liver metastases and primary liver cancers.[44–46] However, the need for an open operation through a midline or subcostal incision and the associated surgical morbidity are the major disadvantages with HAI pump placement. This weakness can be circumvented with robotic placement of the infusion pump.

HAI pump has been placed successfully with laparoscopic techniques but requires a high level of laparoscopic skills.[47,48] The use of long instruments with amplification of hand tremor, only 4° of motion, and a 2-dimensional operative field view makes the required meticulous dissection of the hepatic artery demanding and difficult. Advancement of the catheter in the gastroduodenal artery is especially challenging because of the fulcrum effect. The robotic platform imparts improved depth perception secondary to magnified 3-dimensional view, negated hand tremor, and enhanced manual dexterity, giving the surgeon an unparalleled level of precision and control to perform dissection with finesse. Accurate arteriotomy and intracorporeal suturing are key components of this procedure as well as for advancement of the cannula through the arteriotomy and have been successfully performed and reported.[49]

UNIVERSITY-OF-PITTSBURGH EXPERIENCE WITH ROBOTIC LIVER SURGERY

Since 2007, we have been performing complex surgical oncology procedures with the robot. Our experience now includes more than 150 procedures, including liver resections, bile duct resections, pancreaticoduodenectomies, distal pancreatectomies, total and partial gastrectomies, adrenalectomies, colectomies, low anterior resections, abdominoperineal resections, oophorectomies, hysterectomies, and retroperitoneal tumor resections. Although these procedures are also performed with straight laparoscopy, we prefer the robotic instruments, especially when complex suturing is required or when visibility is difficult, such as with the deep pelvis. The lack

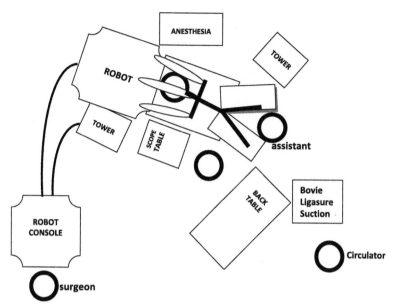

Fig. 3. The operating room schematic for liver surgery.

of tactile feedback is not a significant drawback because the visual cues are extremely strong, but the most significant disadvantages are the setup time and the need for a skilled assistant at the table.

We have performed 15 liver resections (including 1 right hepatic lobectomy, 1 caudate lobectomy, left lateral sectionectomies, complex segmentectomies, and wedge excisions), more than 30 hepaticojejunostomies, and 3 hepatic arterial infusion pump implants. The patient is positioned supine on a split-leg table, with the table in reverse Trendelenburg position. It is helpful to have the table, robotic arms, anesthesia, and nursing carefully arranged from the beginning to avoid delays while docking. A typical operating room setup is demonstrated in **Fig. 3**.

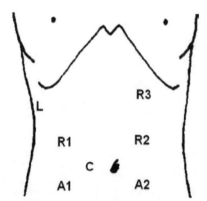

Fig. 4. The recommended port site location for hepatic resections. These ports can be rotated to the patient's right for right-sided wedge resections. A, assistant ports; C, camera ports; L, optional liver retractor; R, robotic ports.

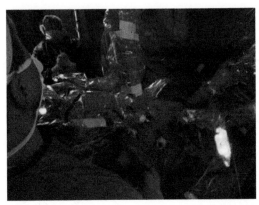

Fig. 5. Assistant surgeon standing between the patient's legs and using the assistant ports during the operation.

The patient is first explored laparoscopically, and ultrasonography of the liver is performed to ensure the feasibility of resection. Three robotic arm ports and a camera port are inserted as demonstrated in **Fig. 4**. The assistant ports are placed inferiorly, and the assistant stands between the split legs (**Fig. 5**). An additional liver retractor port can be placed if needed. The ports can be rotated depending on the location of the resection. We generally perform the liver mobilization and division of the triangular ligament and peritoneal attachments laparoscopically, which sometimes requires movement of the camera port higher in the abdomen and this flexibility is better performed laparoscopically. The need for a hand assist is not necessary, but the tumor margins must be carefully outlined and constantly reexamined with the intraoperative ultrasound.

The robot is then brought to the field and docked. The portal dissection can be performed using the hook cautery, a Maryland dissector, and standard grasping instruments (**Fig. 6**). We use a combination of robotic monopolar cautery, bipolar cautery, and a cauterizing dissecting device handled by the assistant surgeon. The main portal vein branches are divided with the endovascular stapler, and robotic

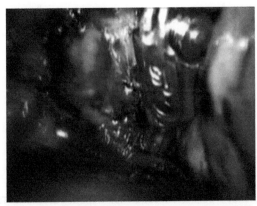

Fig. 6. Robotic isolation of the right hepatic artery in the porta hepatis using the Maryland dissector.

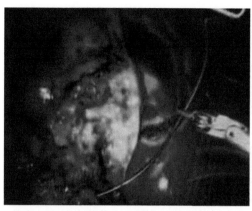

Fig. 7. Robotic placement of large chromic retracting sutures.

locking clips are used for the artery and bile ducts. These can easily be reinforced with silk ties or sutures. The hepatic veins can be dissected extrahepatically or intrahepatically. We have performed both procedures and found that, as with open liver resection, each case has different issues that need to be considered. We use large chromic sutures through the liver for retraction (**Fig. 7**). These sutures can be held by the robot's third arm and greatly aid in the parenchymal dissection by opening the dissection plane. The capsule of the liver is divided with the hook cautery, and parenchymal dissection is accomplished using a crush technique with robotic dissectors (**Figs. 8** and **9**). Small vessels are controlled with bipolar cautery, whereas larger vessels are isolated and clipped, tied, or sutured. Large pedicles or hepatic veins are carefully isolated using robotic dissection, then stapled with an endovascular stapler through the assistant port. It is helpful to have silk and Prolene sutures loaded and ready to pass, in case of bleeding during the parenchymal dissection. The enhanced range of motion achieved with the robotic instruments allow for easy suturing and tying within the parenchyma.

For hepaticojejunostomies, we generally perform the Roux-en-Y anastomosis

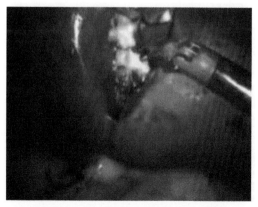

Fig. 8. Robotic incision of the liver capsule using the hook cautery.

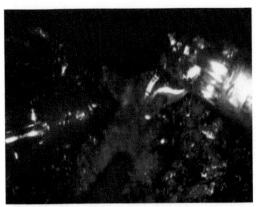

Fig. 9. Robotic parenchymal dissection using a crush technique with the Maryland dissector and bipolar cautery. The assistant uses the suction to keep the field dry.

laparoscopically and place the end of the jejunum through the transverse colon mesentery before docking the robot. This operation can be performed quickly and

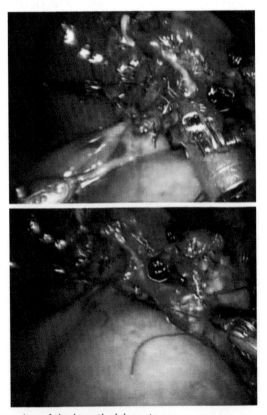

Fig. 10. Robotic suturing of the hepaticojejunostomy.

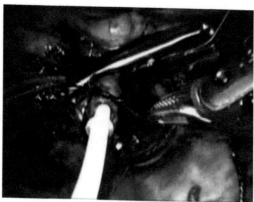

Fig. 11. Robotic placement of the hepatic arterial catheter connected to an infusion pump.

easily laparoscopically using stapling devices without the need for suturing. The robot is then docked and the resection performed. The anastomosis is performed as we do open procedures, with a running posterior layer and an interrupted anterior layer (**Fig. 10**). Corner stitches are placed first and can be held by the third robotic arm for improved visualization. The time efficiency of this anastomosis greatly depends on the skill of the assistant and operating room technician in passing and cutting suture. The hepatic arterial pump insertions are performed exactly as for open procedures. We use small vascular clamps that can be placed with laparoscopic instruments and adjusted with the robotic instruments. Advancing the pump catheter using the robotic arms is much easier than in the straight laparoscopic approach, as is tying the holding sutures around the catheter and vessel (**Fig. 11**).

SUMMARY

Surgery of the liver has progressed tremendously because of a clearer understanding of its functional anatomy, improved knowledge of its regenerative capability, and its functional reserve. Better patient staging and selection, as a result of significant advances in imaging technology, have had a profound effect on the safety of major hepatic resection. Improved techniques to achieve vascular control and technological advancements have facilitated parenchymal transection, resulting in decreased mortality and morbidity from liver surgery. All of this knowledge and technology has been used to extend the scope of liver surgery to incorporate minimally invasive techniques (laparoscopic and robotic) to practically all types of hepatic resections. In addition to the advantages of laparoscopic liver surgery, robotic surgery offers improved visualization and enhanced functionality and maneuverability, thus extending the horizon of minimally invasive liver surgery. The development of new sophisticated surgical robots that are smaller, cheaper, more streamlined, and with tactile feedback, will make robotic surgery more common and popular for these kinds of complex procedures.

In the beginning of the twentieth century, fear of uncontrollable bleeding and friability of the liver parenchyma made the surgeons shy away from open liver surgery; the very same reasons are the grounds for surgeons' hesitance to perform minimally invasive surgery on the liver today. Liver surgery has advanced remarkably and will continue to do so. As in the words of Fortner and Blumgart[50] "It is well to remember that, in the 19th century, surgery was thought to have reached its apogee – but the best is yet to come."

REFERENCES

1. Jones DB, Provost DA, DeMaria EJ, et al. Optimal management of the morbidly obese patient. SAGES appropriateness conference statement. Surg Endosc 2004;18(7): 1029–37.
2. Katkhouda N, Mason RJ, Towfigh S, et al. Laparoscopic versus open appendectomy: a prospective randomized double-blinded study. Ann Surg 2005;242(3):439–48.
3. Hewett PJ, Allardyce RA, Bagshaw PF, et al. Short-term outcomes of the Australian randomized clinical study comparing laparoscopic and conventional open surgical treatments for colon cancer: the ALCCaS trial. Ann Surg 2008;248(5):728–38.
4. Cadiere GB, Himpens J, Germay O, et al. Feasibility of robotic laparoscopic surgery: 146 cases. World J Surg 2001;25(11):1467–77.
5. Berguer R, Rab GT, Abu-Ghaida H, et al. A comparison of surgeon's posture during laparoscopic and open surgical procedures. Surg Endosc 1997;11(2):139–42.
6. Ballantyne GH. The pitfalls of laparoscopic surgery: challenges for robotics and telerobotic surgery. Surg Laparosc Endosc Percutan Tech 2002;12(1):1–5.
7. Cusick RA, Waldhausen JH. The learning curve associated with pediatric laparoscopic splenectomy. Am J Surg 2001;181(5):393–7.
8. Koffron AJ, Auffenberg G, Kung R, et al. Evaluation of 300 minimally invasive liver resections at a single institution: less is more. Ann Surg 2007;246(3):385–92.
9. Gamblin TC, Holloway SE, Heckman JT, et al. Laparoscopic resection of benign hepatic cysts: a new standard. J Am Coll Surg 2008;207(5):731–6.
10. Gayet B, Cavaliere D, Vibert E, et al. Totally laparoscopic right hepatectomy. Am J Surg 2007;194(5):685–9.
11. O'Rourke N, Fielding G. Laparoscopic right hepatectomy: surgical technique. J Gastrointest Surg 2004;8(2):213–6.
12. Nguyen KT, Gamblin TC, Geller DA. World review of laparoscopic liver resection-2,804 patients. Ann Surg 2009;250(5):831–41.
13. Dagher I, O'Rourke N, Geller DA, et al. Laparoscopic major hepatectomy: an evolution in standard of care. Ann Surg 2009;250(5):856–60.
14. Farges O, Jagot P, Kirstetter P, et al. Prospective assessment of the safety and benefit of laparoscopic liver resections. J Hepatobiliary Pancreat Surg 2002;9(2):242–8.
15. Huscher CG, Lirici MM, Chiodini S. Laparoscopic liver resections. Semin Laparosc Surg 1998;5(3):204–10.
16. Lesurtel M, Cherqui D, Laurent A, et al. Laparoscopic versus open left lateral hepatic lobectomy: a case-control study. J Am Coll Surg 2003;196(2):236–42.
17. Hanley EJ, Talamini MA. Robotic abdominal surgery. Am J Surg 2004;188(19S–26.
18. Delaney CP, Lynch AC, Senagore AJ, et al. Comparison of robotically performed and traditional laparoscopic colorectal surgery. Dis Colon Rectum 2003;46(12):1633–9.
19. Anvari M, Birch DW, Bamehriz F, et al. Robotic-assisted laparoscopic colorectal surgery. Surg Laparosc Endosc Percutan Tech 2004;14(6):311–5.
20. Ahlering TE, Skarecky D, Lee D, et al. Successful transfer of open surgical skills to a laparoscopic environment using a robotic interface: initial experience with laparoscopic radical prostatectomy. J Urol 2003;170(5):1738–41.
21. Berryhill R Jr, Jhaveri J, Yadav R, et al. Robotic prostatectomy: a review of outcomes compared with laparoscopic and open approaches. Urology 2008;72(1):15–23.
22. Buell JF, Cherqui D, Geller DA, et al. The international position on laparoscopic liver surgery: the Louisville statement, 2008. Ann Surg 2009;250(5):825–30.

23. Boggi U, Moretto C, Vistoli F, et al. Robotic suture of a large caval injury caused by endo-GIA stapler malfunction during laparoscopic wedge resection of liver segments VII and VIII en-bloc with the right hepatic vein. Minim Invasive Ther Allied Technol 2009;11–5.

24. Choi SB, Park JS, Kim JK, et al. Early experiences of robotic-assisted laparoscopic liver resection. Yonsei Med J 2008;49(4):632–8.

25. Vasile S, Sgarbură O, Tomulescu V, et al. The robotic-assisted left lateral hepatic segmentectomy: the next step. Chirurgia 2008;103(4):401–5.

26. Kang CM, Chi HS, Kim JY, et al. A case of robot-assisted excision of choledochal cyst, hepaticojejunostomy, and extracorporeal Roux-en-y anastomosis using the da Vinci surgical system. Surg Laparosc Endosc Percutan Tech 2007;17(6):538–41.

27. Meehan JJ, Elliott S, Sandler A. The robotic approach to complex hepatobiliary anomalies in children: preliminary report. J Pediatr Surg 2007;42(12):2110–4.

28. Woo R, Le D, Albanese CT, et al. Robot-assisted laparoscopic resection of a type I choledochal cyst in a child. J Laparoendosc Adv Surg Tech A 2006;16(2):179–83.

29. Farello GA, Cerofolini A, Rebonato M, et al. Congenital choledochal cyst: video-guided laparoscopic treatment. Surg Laparosc Endosc 1995;5(5):354–8.

30. Weiss L, Grandmann E, Torhost J, et al. Hematogenous metastatic patterns in colonic carcinoma: an analysis of 1541 necropsies. J Pathol 1986;150(3):195–203.

31. Fong YC, Fortner AM, Enker JG, et al. Liver resection for colorectal metastases. J Clin Oncol 1997;15(3):938–46.

32. Nordlinger B, Guiguet M, Vaillant JC, et al. Surgical resection of colorectal carcinoma metastases to the liver. A prognostic scoring system to improve case selection, based on 1568 patients. Association Francaise de Chirurgie. Cancer 1996;77(7):1254–62.

33. Adam R. Colorectal cancer with synchronous liver metastases. Br J Surg 2007;94(2): 129–31.

34. Capussotti L, Ferrero A, Vigano L, et al. Major liver resections synchronous with colorectal surgery. Ann Surg Oncol 2007;14(1):195–201.

35. The Clinical Outcomes of Surgical Therapy Study Group A comparison of laparo-scopically assisted and open colectomy for colon cancer. N Engl J Med 2004; 350(20):2050–9.

36. Jayne DG, Guillou PJ, Thorpe H, et al. Randomized trial of laparoscopic-assisted resection of colorectal carcinoma: 3-year results of the UK MRC CLASICC Trial Group. J Clin Oncol 2007;25(21):3061–8.

37. Patriti A, Ceccarelli G, Bartoli A, et al. Laparoscopic and robot-assisted one-stage resection of colorectal cancer with synchronous liver metastases: a pilot study. J Hepatobiliary Pancreat Surg 2009;16(4):450–7.

38. Endo I, Gonen M, Yopp AC, et al. Intrahepatic cholangiocarcinoma: rising frequency, improved survival, and determinants of outcome after resection. Ann Surg 2008; 248(1):1–13.

39. Fong Y, Sun RL, Jarnagin W, et al. An analysis of 412 cases of hepatocellular carcinoma at a Western center. Ann Surg 1999;229(6):790–9.

40. Knox JJ, Hedley D, Oza A, et al. Combining gemcitabine and capecitabine in patients with advanced biliary cancer: a phase II trial. J Clin Oncol 2005;23(10):2332–8.

41. Andre T, Tournigand C, Rosmorduc O, et al. Gemcitabine combined with oxaliplatin (GEMOX) in advanced biliary tract adenocarcinoma: a GERCOR study. Ann Oncol 2004;15(9):1339–43.

42. Abou-Alfa GK, Schwartz L, Ricci S, et al. Phase II study of sorafenib in patients with advanced hepatocellular carcinoma. J Clin Oncol 2006;24(26):4293–300.

43. Ong ES, Poirier M, Espat NJ. Hepatic intra-arterial chemotherapy. Ann Surg Oncol 2006;13(2):142–9.

44. Kemeny N, Huang Y, Cohen AM, et al. Hepatic arterial infusion of chemotherapy after resection of hepatic metastases from colorectal cancer. N Engl J Med 1999;341(27): 2039–48.

45. Kemeny MM, Adak S, Gray B, et al. Combined-modality treatment for resectable metastatic colorectal carcinoma to the liver: surgical resection of hepatic metastases in combination with continuous infusion of chemotherapy, an intergroup study. J Clin Oncol 2002;20(6):1499–505.

46. Jarnagin WR, Schwartz LH, Gultekin DH, et al. Regional chemotherapy for unresectable primary liver cancer: results of a phase II clinical trial and assessment of DCE-MRI as a biomarker of survival. Ann Oncol 2009;20(9):1589–95.

47. Urbach DR, Herron DM, Khajanchee YS, et al. Laparoscopic hepatic artery infusion pump placement. Arch Surg 2001;136(6):700–4.

48. Franklin ME Jr, Gonzalez JJ Jr. Laparoscopic placement of hepatic artery catheter for regional chemotherapy infusion: technique, benefits, and complications. Surg Laparosc Endosc Percutan Tech 2002;12(6):398–407.

49. Hellan M, Pigazzi A. Robotic-assisted placement of a hepatic artery infusion catheter for regional chemotherapy. Surg Endosc 2008;22(2):548–51.

50. Fortner JG, Blumgart LH. A historic perspective of liver surgery for tumors at the end of the millennium. J Am Coll Surg 2001;193(2):210–22.

Technological Advances in Robotic-Assisted Laparoscopic Surgery

Gerald Y. Tan, MBChB, MRCSEd, MMed, FAMS[a,c], Raj K. Goel, MD, FRCSC[b],
Jihad H. Kaouk, MD[b], Ashutosh K. Tewari, MD, MCh[a],*

KEYWORDS
- Robot • Single-port • NOTES • Haptics • Simulator
- Laparoscopic • Navigation • Telestration

This article is not certified for AMA PRA Category 1 Credit™ because product brand names are included in the educational content. The Accreditation Council for Continuing Medical Education requires the use of generic names and or drug/product classes as the required nomenclature for therapeutic options in continuing medical education.
For more information, please go to www.accme.org and review the Standards of Commercial Support.

Despite its relative infancy, laparoscopic surgery has radically transformed the landscape of operative urology. The advent of surgical robotics at the turn of the new millennium heralded a quantum leap forward for minimally invasive urologists, who first used it successfully for performing robotic-assisted radical prostatectomy. Since then, there has been an unprecedented explosion in the use of robotics in other aspects of oncologic and reconstructive urologic procedures, with more than 55,000 radical prostatectomies performed with da Vinci® (Intuitive Surgical, Inc, Sunnyvale, CA, USA) robotic assistance in the United States in 2007[1] and more than 70,000

A version of this article was previously published in *Urologic Clinics* 36:2.
Dr Tewari has received a research grant from Intuitive Surgical, Inc. Dr Tan receives financial support from the Ferdinand C. Valentine Fellowship in Urologic Research, New York Academy of Medicine and the Medical Research Fellowship, National Medical Research Council, Singapore. Dr Kaouk serves as a proctor for Intuitive Surgical Inc.
 a Brady Foundation, Department of Urology, Weill Medical College of Cornell University, New York Presbyterian Hospital, 525 East 68th Street, Starr 900, New York, NY 10065, USA
b Glickman Urological and Kidney Institute, Cleveland Clinic Foundation, 9500 Euclid Avenue, Cleveland, OH 44195, USA
c Department of Urology, Tan Tock Seng Hospital, 11 Jalan Tan Tock Seng, Singapore 308433, Singapore
* Corresponding author.
E-mail address: ashtewarimd@gmail.com

Perioperative Nursing Clinics 6 (2011) 273–289
doi:10.1016/j.cpen.2011.06.002
1556-7931/11/$ – see front matter © 2011 Elsevier Inc. All rights reserved.
periopnursing.theclinics.com

performed worldwide in 2008 (Intuitive Surgical, Inc, unpublished data, 2008). The increasing popularity of robotic-assisted laparoscopic surgery seems to be mirrored in Europe and other parts of the world, and in the arenas of cardiothoracic, gynecologic, and general surgery.[2–4]

Propelling this zeitgeist for surgical robotics have been exciting advances in robotic technologies and their potential applications in urologic surgery. This article therefore serves as a timely review of these promising innovations to date and discusses likely future directions for our craft as the practice of surgery becomes increasingly robotic-assisted and computer-aided.

EVOLUTION OF UROLOGIC ROBOTIC SYSTEMS AND CURRENT STATE OF THE ART

Urologic robotic systems used in recent years have essentially comprised a computer with real-time imaging capability linked to various effector units for execution of specific tasks. Off-line (ie, fixed path) robots are automated systems that execute precise movements within specified confines based on preprogrammed imaging studies obtained before surgery, operating independently without requiring active input from the surgeon.[5] These include (1) robots for prostate access, such as the ProBot (prototype by a team from Imperial College, London—not commercially available and not manufactured), a robotic resection device with 7 df, and various robotic prostate biopsy systems,[6–8] and (2) renal access systems, such as the PAKY-RCM and Acubot robots (prototypes developed by Stoianovici et al at URobotics Laboratory, Johns Hopkins Medical Institute, Baltimore, MA, USA), for precise percutaneous access to the kidney.[9,10]

Conversely, on-line robotic systems are designed to replicate the surgeon's movements in real time in the operative field with improved tremor-free precision and scale adjustment when applicable. These surgeon-directed robots may be broadly divided into endoscope manipulators and master-slave systems. Endoscopic manipulators, such as the Automated Endoscopic System for Optimal Positioning (AESOP; Intuitive Surgical Inc) and Naviot (Hitachi Hybrid Network Co, Ltd, Yokohama, Japan) systems, have the benefits of being less expensive, smaller, and easier to set up with stable adjustable positioning, but their usefulness remains limited in complex operations.[5] Master-slave systems, such as the now obsolete Zeus (originally manufactured by Computer Motion, Inc, Goleta, CA, USA) and the da Vinci® system, comprise a computerized surgical console connected to an endoscopic manipulator with two or three robotic arms for instrument manipulation. Precise digital control of surgical instruments through the console eliminates movement tremors and allows motion scaling, wherein the surgeon's movements may be amplified or dampened.

The most commercially successful robotic system to date has been the da Vinci® system,[11] with more than 1000 systems currently installed in hospitals worldwide. From its inception, the benefits of the da Vinci® system over conventional laparoscopy were readily apparent: superior ergonomics; optical magnification of the operative field within direct control of the console surgeon; and enhanced dexterity, precision, and control of operative movements. Comprising a patient-side cart with three or four robotic manipulator arms connected to a master console, the da Vinci's binocular images obtained by means of the laparoscopic camera lens (0° or 30°) are integrated by the computer to provide a composite three-dimensional (3D) image when viewed by means of the immersive stereo viewer at the console. The patented robotic instruments also have additional articulating joints (EndoWrist; Intuitive Surgical, Inc) that permit 7 df of movement, empowering the minimally invasive surgeon to perform intracorporeal suturing and dissection intuitively and effortlessly.

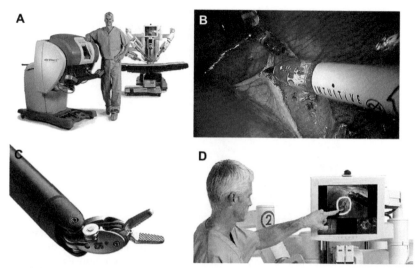

Fig. 1. (A) Surgeon console, patient cart, and robotic arms of the da Vinci® S HD Surgical System. (B) High-resolution 3D real-time images of the operative field as seen through the immersive viewer. (C) EndoWrist capable of 7 df of movement. (D) Interactive Tilepro® integrated touch-screen video display allows telestration and proctoring during live surgery, with multi-input display of a patient's preoperative clinical data and images. (*Courtesy of* Intuitive Surgical, Inc, Sunnyvale, CA; with permission.)

Its current state-of-the-art version, the da Vinci® S HD Surgical System (Intuitive Surgical, Inc), integrates 3D high-definition vision capability with the existing robotic platform, providing twice the effective viewing resolution with improved clarity and detail of tissue planes (**Fig. 1**). Its digital zoom function reduces interference between the endoscope and instruments, and the integrated touch-screen monitor permits telestration for improved proctoring and team communication. In addition, the TilePro® (Intuitive Surgical, Inc) multi-image stereo viewer enables simultaneous display of multiple video inputs in the surgeon console, integrating display of the patient's ultrasound, CT, and MRI images. Extended-reach instruments are also now available for multiquadrant access, with a 50% increase in pitch and yaw range of motion and four times the working volume.[12] Fewer cable connections between components has also helped to shorten setup time, and a high-speed fiberoptic connection in the surgical platform offers the potential for remote telementoring.

Despite these technical innovations, there still exist some limitations. First, the da Vinci® S HD Surgical System is unable to provide haptic feedback for the console surgeon, who must necessarily base his or her intraoperative decisions on visual cues encountered during surgical dissection. Second, the large size of the robot presents some challenges to the operating staff when docking and repositioning the robot during complex procedures. Third, there remains a lack of simulator technologies available to surgeons and residents desiring familiarity with the robotic console, with their options currently limited to attending training courses that are mostly didactic in nature. Finally, the high cost of this technology may limit or slow the adoption of robotic-assisted laparoscopic surgery on a larger scale internationally.

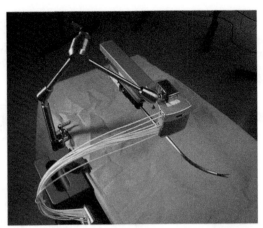

Fig. 2. Photograph of the Laprotek mainframe and guide tube. The stainless-steel guide tube controls upward and downward movement of the instrument, whereas the back end pivots about the incision. The arrow indicates the surgical port site position. (*From* Rentschler ME, Platt SR, Berg K, et al. Miniature in vivo robots for remote and harsh environments. IEEE Trans Inf Technol Biomed 2008;12:66–75; with permission.)

Against this background, we now review some exciting technological advances that promise to redress some of these technical issues and bring the practice of robotic surgery into the mainstream.

MINIATURIZATION OF ROBOTIC PLATFORM

The current design of the da Vinci's robotic cart is based on the traditional laparoscopic platform, wherein straight rigid instruments are used intracorporeally through small incisions by the surgeon maneuvering the instrument handles outside the patient's body. As a result, the current da Vinci® system occupies significant overhead over the sterile field, presenting spatial challenges for the patient-side assistants to overcome to operate dexterously alongside the robotic arms and cart.

In contrast, the Laprotek system (EndoVia, Inc, Norwood, MA, USA subsequently taken over by Hansen Medical, Inc, Mountain View, CA, USA) comprises slave instrument "motor packs" that are mechanically mounted on the existing bed rails of the operating table. The movements from these motors are then transmitted to the surgical instruments by means of stainless-steel cables. Whereas the da Vinci® system directs its straight instruments by moving their back handles through a 3D cone, the Laprotek system uses a curved guide tube to position its instruments intracorporeally. Its design occupies significantly less space in the sterile field, reducing collisions between the robotic instruments and camera (**Fig. 2**). Although not commercially available, it has been projected to cost significantly less than the da Vinci® system.

Working on the premise that the motion outside the patient should be confined to a line rather than a cone (da Vinci® system) or a plane (Laprotek system), Dachs and Peine[13] proposed a new design wherein the robotic instruments would have two movable joints within the body that would permit 6 *df* of movement without requiring corresponding external pivoting motions (**Fig. 3**). Because the instruments would not be constrained to pivot about the port side, they could be easily mounted on a streamlined mechanical arm that supports its linear track to deliver comparable

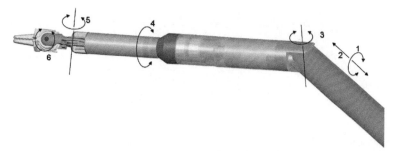

Fig. 3. Pictorial representation of new tool design permitting 6 *df* of movement intracorporeally. (*From* Dachs GW II, Peine WJ. A novel surgical robot design: minimizing the operating envelope within the sterile field. Conf Proc IEEE Eng Med Biol Soc 2006;1:1505–8; with permission. Copyright © 2006 IEEE.)

intracorporeal dexterity and precision. The advantages of their proposed design would include minimization of machinery in the exterior working envelope, giving surgical assistants more room to operate, and elimination of instrument collisions attributable to suboptimal port placement (**Fig. 4**).

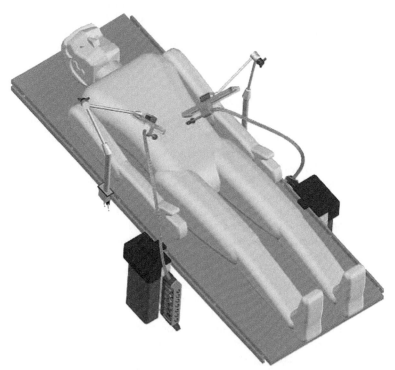

Fig. 4. Envisioned design of robotic setup as proposed by Dachs and Peine. (*From* Dachs GW II, Peine WJ. A novel surgical robot design: minimizing the operating envelope within the sterile field. Conf Proc IEEE Eng Med Biol Soc 2006;1:1505–8; with permission. Copyright © 2006 IEEE.)

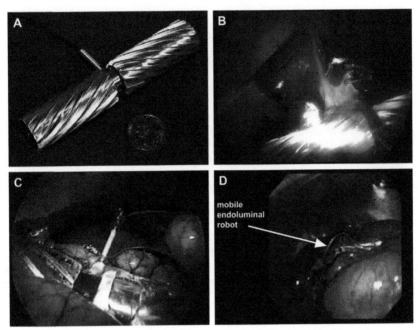

Fig. 5. (A) Mobile adjustable-focus robotic camera (MARC) prototype designed by research-ers at the University of Nebraska. (B) Intracorporeal view of the MARC during porcine cholecystectomy, (C) Mobile in vivo robot executes liver biopsy. (D) Same robot performs peritoneoscopy. (From Oleynikov D. Robotic surgery. Surg Clin North Am 2008;88:1121–30; with permission.)

MOBILE MINIATURIZED IN VIVO ROBOTS

Despite improvements in high-definition real-time clarity of tissue architecture and a wider field of view with the da Vinci® S HD Surgical System, the surgeon's visual and operative fields remain constrained by camera and instrument placement dictated by the entry incisions. To overcome these limitations, Rentschler and Oleynikov's group from the University of Nebraska[2,14] has explored the use of in vivo microrobots. They first reported the use of miniature in vivo adjustable-focus camera wheeled robots to augment visual feedback to surgeons during laparoscopic cholecystectomy in a canine model. Mounted on two helical wheels driven by direct current motors, these microrobots had sufficient traction to move over slick deformable abdominal viscera without causing injury (**Fig. 5**). The same investigators subsequently designed a fixed-base pan-and-tilt camera robot that permitted forward tilting at an angle of 45°. Comprising tripod legs that were spring-loadable and could be abducted during insertion through the laparoscopic port, this microrobot could then be guided into a desired intra-abdominal position with laparoscopic instruments, offering surgeons alternate views of the organs being operated on to that obtained by means of the laparoscopic camera.[15] Joseph and colleagues[16] recently reported their collaborative experience with these prototypes in performing laparoscopic prostatectomy and laparoscopic nephrectomy in a canine model. Rentschler and colleagues[17] also demonstrated their use in guiding a surgically naive crew member to perform the steps of a laparoscopic appendectomy in a harsh environment by means of remote telementoring. Albeit successful, technical drawbacks encountered during these operations included the need for a separate controller to maneuver the robot into position; significant hindrance attributable to the tethered design for the robot's continuous power; and lack of a self-cleaning mechanism for the camera lens positioned between the helical wheels, which resulted in obscured images from direct contact with intra-abdominal organs and fluids.

The feasibility of using multiple miniature in vivo robots for bettering spatial orientation while facilitating tasks was recently reported by Lehman and colleagues.[18] They used three robots—a peritoneum-mounted camera robot, a lighting robot, and a retraction robot—together with a conventional upper gastrointestinal endoscope to augment the scope of natural orifice transluminal endoscopic surgery (NOTES) procedures in a porcine model.

Although still in their early stages, these and other feasibility studies[19–21] have demonstrated significant potential for eventual development of wireless robotic sensors to provide composite all-round real-time images and robotic manipulators that would obviate the need for multiple incision sites for instrument access.

ADVANCES IN ENDOSCOPIC NAVIGATION SYSTEMS

In performing laparoscopic urologic procedures with da Vinci® assistance, surgeons rely on visual cues instead of tactile feedback to achieve comparable outcomes to those reported for traditional open surgery. Suture tension, for example, has been dictated by the degree of deformation on the respective tissue. Imaging technologies based on virtual and augmented reality have evolved to provide real-time navigational guidance for the surgeon to perform image-guided surgery. Augmented reality may be defined as the integration of computer-generated images (from reconstructed preoperative MRI, CT, or ultrasound images) to live video or other real-time images, such as ultrasound, allowing visualization of visceral anatomy and surrounding structures.[22]

The initial experience of such image-guided surgery in neurosurgery, maxillofacial surgery, and orthopedics was based on integrating images over fixed bony landmarks.[23–25] Attempts to extrapolate its use in abdominal surgery have highlighted the challenges of imaging viscera that constantly shifts and undergoes deformation: (1) to find constant intra-abdominal reference points and (2) to merge preoperative images over constantly shifting soft tissue anatomy attributable to breathing, heartbeat, patient movement, and surgical instrumentation.[22,26]

Ukimura and Gill[27] recently described their experience of using a color-coded zonal navigation system to perform laparoscopic partial nephrectomy. Such a system affords the surgeon a 3D visual surgical roadmap based on preoperative CT images to identify safe resection margins during surgery by giving different colors to the tumor and its adjacent tissues. Ukimura and his colleagues[28–30] further reported the use of intraoperative transrectal 3D ultrasonography to guide the course of laparoscopic nerve-sparing radical prostatectomy.

Attempts at incorporating conventional fluoroscopy during robotic procedures have been hindered by spatial difficulties of reconciling the sizable overhead footprint of the fluoroscopic and da Vinci® systems over the sterile field. In addition, fluoroscopy only provides cursory images of calcified or radiopaque structures, with limited soft tissue information; the need for operating staff to wear heavy protective gowns to protect them from collateral radiation exposure is an unattractive prospect during complex laparoscopic procedures; and the anterior-posterior images afforded by fluoroscopy leave many "blind spots" during surgical dissection.[31]

The TilePro® system uses a "picture in picture" viewer in the da Vinci® surgeon's console to toggle among images from various sources. Bhayani and Snow[32] recently described their experience with this system to assimilate images from preoperative CT or MRI scans, real-time ultrasonographic images, and 3D images viewed through the da Vinci® surgeon console during robotic-assisted laparoscopic partial and radical nephrectomy. In 2 of 17 partial nephrectomies, superselective arterial control was possible using Doppler information fed into the surgical console during tumor resection. Although providing invaluable information during surgery, the images were static and not superimposable to the mobile operative field. Although the TilePro® system has increased the availability of anatomic images available to the console surgeon during surgery, the ultimate direction would certainly be to integrate these images in real time onto the operative field as seen through the immersive viewer.

ROBOTIC NATURAL ORIFICE TRANSLUMINAL ENDOSCOPIC SURGERY AND SINGLE-PORT SURGERY

NOTES has made significant advancements since its inception in the late 1990s. Using a natural orifice to conceal surgery has not been a new concept to urology, because transurethral procedures, including cystoscopy, prostatectomy, and ureteroscopy, have been routinely performed through a natural orifice for several decades now. Previous limitations in equipment and technique had daunted minimally invasive surgeons from attempting intraperitoneal procedures through a natural orifice, however. Gettman and colleagues[33] successfully performed the first transvaginal NOTES nephrectomy in a porcine model, using conventional laparoscopic equipment through a single abdominal 5-mm trocar. Single-port NOTES access through transvaginal,[34] transgastric,[35] transvesical,[36,37] and even transcolonic[38,39] routes has now been reported. Nonetheless, NOTES procedures remain limited by the degree of mobility and stability afforded by current endoscopic technologies.

Building on their experience with single-port laparoscopic urologic surgery, Kaouk and his colleagues from the Cleveland Clinic[40–42] recently pioneered the use of the da Vinci® system for natural orifice procedures, first in the porcine model[43] and subsequently in humans.[44] The first technical constraint their group encountered was to overcome the critical distance between robotic arms required for uninterrupted maneuverability during surgery. Second, traditional transabdominal placement of robotic trocars creates a fulcrum at the fascial level, allowing the robotic system to recognize a pivot around which the robotic arm can rotate. Altering the ideal location of this fulcrum and constricting port placement potentially predispose to inadvertent tissue injury and restricted movement.

Despite these limitations, configuring the robotic arms in unorthodox positions provided an opportunity to explore the potential of robotics in NOTES. Box and colleagues[39] successfully completed a robotic NOTES porcine nephrectomy by placing the robotic scope through a single abdominal trocar site while the right and left arms of the robot were placed transvaginally and transcolonically, respectively. Given the configuration, the robotic camera required manual control, whereas the robotic arms were manipulated by the surgeon at the console. The porcine nephrectomy was completed uneventfully despite the expected clashing of robotic arms externally. In contrast, Kaouk and colleagues placed the robotic camera lens and one arm through the umbilicus, with the other robotic arm inserted through the vagina, permitting successful completion of more than 30 robotic NOTES procedures to date. The arm configuration provided for greater articulation and closely mimicked internal triangulation as appreciated during standard laparoscopy. In all, robotic NOTES dismembered pyeloplasty, partial nephrectomy, and completion nephrectomy were successfully performed.[43]

Immense interest recently in laparoscopic single-port surgery has also witnessed the emergence of urologic procedures being accomplished through a single multi-channel port.[45–48] As in NOTES, critical analysis of surgical technique identified limitations of the da Vinci® system in instrumentation and dissecting capabilities in such a confined space, chiefly that the proximity of robotic arms through a single multichannel port would invariably lead to external clashing. Attempting novel modifications to port and robotic instrument configuration, Kaouk and colleagues[44] reported the first successful series of single-port robotic procedures in humans, including radical prostatectomy, dismembered pyeloplasty, and radical nephrectomy. A salient highlight of these procedures was the improved facility for intracorporeal dissecting and suturing. During urethral-vesical anastomosis and ureteropelvic anastomosis, a continuous running suture creating a watertight closure was possible because of greater instrument articulation and rigidity.

ADVANCES IN FLEXIBLE ROBOTICS

Abbott and colleagues[49] from Purdue University have been working to develop an endoluminal robotic system (ERS) comprising a camera lens with two adjacent robotic instruments, each having at least 6 df plus an end-effector gripping action. The first-generation design, the ViaCath system (EndoVia Medical, Norwood, MA, USA), was fashioned on the Laprotek master console with haptic interfaces and flexible robotic instruments that run alongside a standard gastroscope or colonoscope. The key components of these robotic instruments are a mechanical coupler to the position arm, a flexible shaft, and an articulating tip with an end effector delivering a total of 7 df within the scope's visual field (**Fig. 6**). The early results in an in vivo porcine model revealed various technical difficulties, chiefly difficulty in intubating the patient and positioning the instruments at the desired site, the instruments catching on tissue during deployment, and the limited lateral force produced by the instruments being insufficient for effectively executing the intended procedures on gastrointestinal tissue. To redress these limitations, the investigators have proposed a second-generation flexible ERS and instruments to improve kinematic instrument control and reduce inherent friction to boost the force available for instrument actuation and manipulation.

Apart from laparoscopic and intraperitoneal procedures, flexible robotic systems have also been applied during ureterorenoscopy. A novel device created by Hansen Medical, Inc incorporates a robotic console to manipulate and control the deflection of a flexible ureteroscope (**Fig. 7**). Using this novel remote system, retrograde ureterorenoscopy was successfully performed in a swine model.[50,51] The increasing range of motion and stability of the platform parallel that of laparoscopic robotic systems. Further refinements in the product may ease the learning curve required during flexible upper tract ureterorenoscopy.

ADVANCES IN HAPTICS

Despite affording the surgeon improved operative dexterity and optical magnification, the current da Vinci® system is unable to deliver the element of haptics. Haptics has been categorized by Okamura[52] as being kinesthetic (involving forces and positions of the muscles and joints) or cutaneous (tactile, related to skin), encompassing the spectrum of force, distributed pressure, temperature, vibrations, and texture. The sense of touch has long been considered essential in limiting inadvertent tissue injury during surgical procedures. Haptics in robotics has demonstrable benefits in reducing tissue injury and reducing suture breakage while maintaining respectable operative time in the hands of an experienced surgeon.[53–57]

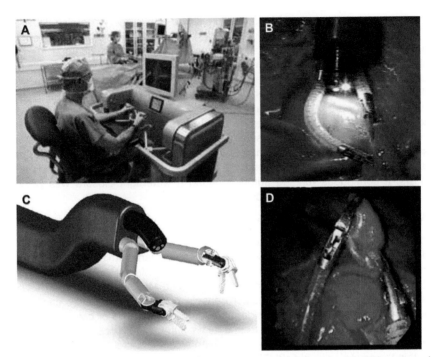

Fig. 6. The ViaCath system. (*A*) Laprotek surgeon console drives the ViaCath system. (*B*) ViaCath instruments use a double-flex section design at the distal tip for articulation. (*C*) Articulated overtube facilitates introduction of the flexible endoscope with its two highly articulated instruments. (*D*) In vivo visualization of abdominal viscera in a porcine model. (*From* Abbott DJ, Becke C, Rothstein RI, et al. Design of an endolumenal NOTES robotic system. In: Proceedings of the IEEE/RSJ International Conference on Intelligent Robots and Systems. San Diego, CA: October 29-November 2, 2007. p. 412; with permission.)

Attempts at developing sensory information from the robotic end effectors are cursory at this time and are largely focused on force-feedback systems. Although successfully used in various engineering situations, the translation of current commercial force-feedback sensors to live surgery has been hampered by constraints in size, design, cost, compatibility, and ability to withstand conventional sterilization procedures. Preliminary evidence that haptic feedback with robotics is possible has emerged, wherein specialized grippers are attached to the jaws of existing robotic instruments to deliver haptic feedback.[57,58] Redesigning robotic instruments to integrate force-sensing capability has also been reported but has not been met with much enthusiasm, given the recurrent prohibitive costs of disposing of these surgical expendables after each case in current practice.

Robotic haptic technology has also found new use in the arena of disaster and emergency medicine.[59] Robotics used for hazardous waste identification and removal has removed individuals from danger by means of direct exposure. These "hazbot" platforms with haptics have demonstrated greater reproducibility and ease of use with novice manipulators. Comparative evaluation between standard robotic systems and more refined humanistic platforms may propel robotics to a new level to improve surgeon ability further.

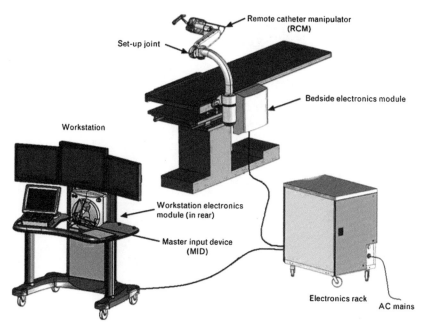

Fig. 7. Pictorial illustration of the flexible robotic catheter-control system. AC, alternating current. (*Courtesy of* Hansen Medical, Mountain View, CA; © 2009 Hansen Inc. Used with permission.)

ADVANCES IN SIMULATOR TRAINING PLATFORMS FOR ROBOTICS

Another significant hurdle in assimilating robotics into the vanguard of mainstream urologic surgery involves the training of robotic-naive surgeons with no prior experience at the robotic console. The high costs of purchasing and housing a dedicated dry laboratory "training" da Vinci® system and the cost of surgical expendables used during training cases in wet laboratories often mean that console experience obtained at various hands-on courses is limited and fleetingly transient. In addition, heightened expectations from patients undergoing robotic surgery, medicolegal implications of accountability of attending surgeons, and demands from hospital administrators to turn around robotic procedures have resulted in limited opportunities for urology residents to gain operative maturity at the console.

The dV-Trainer (MIMIC Technologies, Inc, Seattle, WA, USA) has been developed in collaboration with Intuitive Surgical, Inc as a solution to some of these current obstacles in surgical training.[60,61] It consists of a master console with finger-cuff telemanipulators connected to a binocular 3D visual output that aims to reproduce the look and feel of the da Vinci® console. The program encompasses exercises in EndoWrist manipulation, camera control, clutching, object transfer and placement, needle handling, needle driving, knot tying, and suturing. The cable-driven system also provides haptic feedback for the trainee as he or she executes surgical movements spatially (**Fig. 8**). Among 15 subjects with varying experience with robotic surgery, Lendvay and colleagues[62] reported significant reduction of total task time, economy of motion, and time the telemanipulators spent outside of the center of the platform's workspace in the experienced group compared with the novice group.

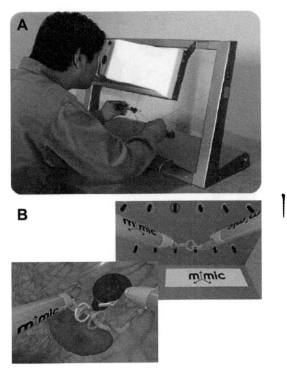

Fig. 8. The dV-Trainer. (*A*) Binocular console with 3D image viewer. (*B*) Virtual reality images seen through the viewer. (*Courtesy of* MIMIC Technologies, Seattle, WA; with permission.)

Researchers at the University of Nebraska are also working to produce a da Vinci®-compatible virtual reality simulator, using kinematic data from the da Vinci® console through LabVIEW (National Instruments, Austin, TX, USA) to drive simulation software (Cyberbotics, Ltd, Lausanne, Switzerland).[63,64] Medical Education Technologies, Inc (Sarasota, FL, USA) has also made an attempt to produce a robotic surgery simulator for its SurgicalSIM package,[65] although the reception to this has yet to be reported.

ADVANCES IN REMOTE ROBOTIC SURGERY

In 2001, Marescaux and colleagues[66] reported the first experience of performing transatlantic robotic-assisted laparoscopic cholecystectomies in six pigs and one human, with the surgeon based in New York and the Zeus system installed in Strasbourg, France. Anvari and colleagues[67] subsequently reported their experience of 21 telerobotic laparoscopic operations between St Joseph's Hospital in Hamilton, Ontario, Canada and North Bay General Hospital 400 km north of Hamilton. Through an IP-VPN (15 Mbps of bandwidth) network that linked the Zeus robotic console in the teaching institute with the three arms of the Zeus TS System (Computer Motion Inc, Santa Barbara, CA, USA) in the rural hospital, the surgeons were able to operate together with the same surgical footprint, with overall latency at 135 to 140 milliseconds.[67] Their experience, albeit with two-dimensional vision, demonstrated the huge potential of robotic platforms to deliver care in remote areas and combat situations, in addition to telestrating complex robotic-assisted laparoscopic procedures to surgeons on the learning curve.

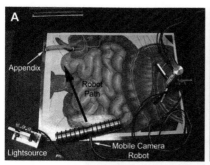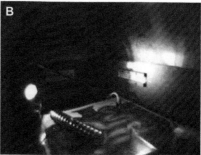

Fig. 9. (*A*) Setup for telementoring of the surgically naive crew of the NEEMO 9 mission to perform a simple appendectomy. (*B*) Real-time visual feedback of the appendectomy by means of the mobile robot's adjustable camera. (*From* Rentschler ME, Platt SR, Berg K, et al. Miniature in vivo robots for remote and harsh environments. IEEE Trans Inf Technol Biomed 2008;12:66–75; with permission.)

Sterbis and colleagues[68] recently reported the first experience with transcontinental robotic surgery using the da Vinci® system. Video and robotic signals were transmitted over the Internet using nondedicated lines and commercial video coding and decoding systems (Plycom, Pleasanton, CA, USA and Haivision, Montreal, Quebec, Canada). This enabled surgeons at two separate consoles (1300 and 2400 miles away from the robot, respectively) to control different parts of the same robot to complete four nephrectomies in a porcine model successfully. The round-trip delay of 900 milliseconds using a bandwidth of 3 Mbps resulted in intermittently poor vision, whereas the second console surgeon using a bandwidth of 8 Mbps had good visualization throughout with a latency of 450 milliseconds (with the difference in bandwidth being attributable to the 3D instead of two-dimensional images being transmitted).

The University of Nebraska team also recently reported the feasibility of telementoring the crew of the National Aeronautics and Space Administration (NASA) Extreme Environment Mission Operations (NEEMO) 9 mission in executing the steps of a laparoscopic appendectomy using these in vivo microrobots.[17] In this study, the crew member was telementored by means of video conferencing software after viewing a 30-second video describing the steps of the appendectomy and successfully dissected, stapled, and removed the appendix (**Fig. 9**). Lum and colleagues[69] from the University of Washington also reported their experience with the RAVEN robot (prototype designed by Dr Blake Hannaford and his team from the Biorobotics Laboratory, Department of Electrical Engineering, University of Washington, Seattle, Washington—not yet commercially available), a prototype smaller in size than the da Vinci® system with the capability of being mounted on the patient and operated in harsh and remote environments (**Fig. 10**). Bell and colleagues[70] from the same institute also reported on their experience with a brain-computer interface that allows a person to control a humanoid robot directly using noninvasive brain signals from the scalp through electroencephalography. In that study, a partially autonomous robot was able to perform complex tasks like walking to specific locations and picking up specific objects under direction from nine different users.

As rapid advances in Internet technologies for swifter and more secure transmission of data couple the developments in surgical robotics, it is foreseeable that robotic telestration and remote surgery are likely to become commonplace practices in the not too distant future, possibly even with hands-off control of advanced robotic instruments.

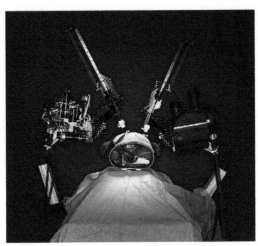

Fig. 10. The RAVEN robot designed at the University of Washington. (*From* Oleynikov D. Robotic surgery. Surg Clin North Am 2008;88:1121–30; with permission.)

SUMMARY

The advent of novel robotic and compatible technologies has occurred at a breathtaking pace in the past decade, mirroring the rapid adoption of robotic surgery among urologists and their patients worldwide. The current da Vinci® S HD System represents the state of the art, incorporating several new features that have made surgery more ergonomic and interactive for console surgeons and their patient-side assistants. Early trials of micro-electrical mechanical systems devices have been encouraging, and the next step would be to refine these technologies further for empowering the surgeon with augmented real-time visualization of tissue and intracorporeal dexterity, possibly even through a single port. Virtual reality simulator training packages compatible with the da Vinci® system are going to be commercially available soon, giving robotically naive surgeons a much needed bridge for gaining familiarity and confidence at the console before live surgery. Image-guided surgery should also become increasingly more popular as technologies develop to overcome the current limitations of working with deformable mobile viscera. Developments in data and image transmission over Internet protocols and satellite platforms may soon allow remote telestration of complex robotic operations, obviating the need for surgeons to be physically present to perform or mentor such operations and delivering improved patient care to those living in remote or hazardous environments. These promising innovations look set to usher in a new era in operative urology in the near future, and the authors look forward with immense interest to how this article may be deemed archaic in a few years.

ACKNOWLEDGMENTS

The authors thank the management of Intuitive Surgical, Inc (Sunnyvale, CA, USA) and MIMIC Technologies (Seattle, WA, USA) for their invaluable constructive input and use of their illustrations for this article.

REFERENCES

1. Su L. Role of robotics in modern urologic practice. Curr Opin Urol 2009;19:63–4.
2. Oleynikov D. Robotic surgery. Surg Clin North Am 2008;88:1121–30.

3. Stoianovici D. Robotic surgery. World J Urol 2000;18:289–95.
4. Camarillo DB, Krummel TM, Salisbury K. Robotic technology in surgery: past, present and future. Am J Surg 2004;188:2S–15.
5. Sim HG, Yip SKH, Cheng CWS. Equipment and technology in surgical robotics. World J Urol 2006;24:128–35.
6. Harris SJ, Arambula-Cosio F, Mei Q, et al. The Probot—an active robot for prostate resection. Proc Inst Mech Eng [H] 1997;211:317–25.
7. Rovetta A, Sala R. Execution of robot-assisted biopsies within the clinical context. J Image Guid Surg 1995;1:280–7.
8. Hempel E, Fischer H, Gumb L, et al. An MRI-compatible surgical robot for precise radiological interventions. Comput Aided Surg 2003;8:180–91.
9. Cadeddu JA, Bzotek A, Schreiner S, et al. A robotic system for percutaneous renal access. J Urol 1997;158:1589–93.
10. Cleary K, Melzer A, Watson V, et al. Interventional robotic systems: applications and technology state-of-the-art. Minim Invasive Ther Allied Technol 2006;15:101–13.
11. Mozer P, Troccaz J, Stoianovici D. Urologic robots and future directions. Curr Opin Urol 2009;19:114–9.
12. Available at: www.intuitivesurgical.com/products/davincissurgicalsystem. Accessed March 23, 2009.
13. Dachs GW II, Peine WJ. A novel surgical robot design: minimizing the operating envelope within the sterile field. Conf Proc IEEE Eng Med Biol Soc 2006;1:1505–8.
14. Rentschler ME, Dumpert J, Platt SR, et al. Mobile in vivo camera robots provide sole visual feedback for abdominal exploration and cholecystectomy. Surg Endosc 2006; 20:135–8.
15. Rentschler ME, Oleynikov D. Recent in vivo surgical robot and mechanism developments. Surg Endosc 2007;21:1477–81.
16. Joseph JV, Oleynikov D, Rentschler ME, et al. Microrobot assisted laparoscopic urological surgery in a canine model. J Urol 2008;180:2202–5.
17. Rentschler ME, Platt SR, Berg K, et al. Miniature in vivo robots for remote and harsh environments. IEEE Trans Inf Technol Biomed 2008;12:66–75.
18. Lehman AC, Berg KA, Dumpert J, et al. Surgery with cooperative robots. Comput Aided Surg 2008;13:95–105.
19. Hawks JA, Rentschler ME, Redden L, et al. Towards an in vivo wireless mobile robot for surgical assistance. Stud Health Technol Inform 2008;132:153–8.
20. Rentschler ME, Dumpert J, Platt SR, et al. Mobile in vivo biopsy and camera robot. Stud Health Technol Inform 2006;119:449–54.
21. Rentschler ME, Dumpert J, Platt SR, et al. Natural orifice surgery with an endoluminal mobile robot. Surg Endosc 2007;21:1212–5.
22. Teber D, Baumhauer M, Guven EO, et al. Robotic and imaging in urological surgery. Curr Opin Urol 2009;19:108–13.
23. Fox WC, Warzyniak S, Chandler WF. Intraoperative acquisition of three-dimensional imaging for frameless stereotactic guidance during transsphenoidal pituitary surgery using the Arcadis Orbic System. J Neurosurg 2008;108:746–50.
24. Tian Z, Lu W, Wang T, et al. Application of a robotic telemanipulation system in stereotactic surgery. Stereotact Funct Neurosurg 2008;86:54–61.
25. Paul HA, Bargner WL, Mittelstadt B, et al. Development of a surgical robot for cementless hip arthroplasty. Clin Orthop 1992;285:57–66.
26. Baumhauer M, Feuerstein M, Meinzer HP, et al. Navigation in endoscopic soft tissue surgery: perspectives and limitations. J Endourol 2008;22:751–66.
27. Ukimura O, Gill IS. Imaging assisted endoscopic surgery: Cleveland Clinic experience. J Endourol 2008;22:803–10.

28. Ukimura O, Magi-Galluzzi C, Gill IS. Real-time transrectal ultrasound guidance during laparoscopic radical prostatectomy: impact on surgical margins. J Urol 2006;175: 1304–10.

29. Ukimura O, Gill IS. Real-time transrectal ultrasound guidance during nerve-sparing laparoscopic radical prostatectomy: pictorial essay. J Urol 2006;175:1311–9.

30. Ukimura O, Ahlering TE, Gill IS. Transrectal ultrasound-guided, energy-free, nerve-sparing laparoscopic radical prostatectomy. J Endourol 2008;22:1993–5.

31. Afthinos JN, Latif MJ, Bhora FY, et al. What technical barriers exist for real time fluoroscopic and video image overlay in robotic surgery? Int J Med Robot 2008;4: 368–72.

32. Bhayani SB, Snow DC. Novel dynamic information integration during da Vinci robotic partial nephrectomy and radical nephrectomy. Journal of Robotic Surgery 2008;2: 67–9.

33. Gettman MT, Lotan Y, Napper CA, et al. Transvaginal laparoscopic nephrectomy: development and feasibility in the porcine model. Urology 2002;59:446–50.

34. Clayman RV, Box GN, Abraham JB, et al. Rapid communication: transvaginal single-port NOTES nephrectomy: initial laboratory experience. J Endourol 2007;21: 640–4.

35. Kalloo AN, Singh VK, Jagannath SB, et al. Flexible transgastric peritoneoscopy: a novel approach to diagnostic and therapeutic interventions in the peritoneal cavity. Gastrointest Endosc 2004;60:114–7.

36. Lima E, Rolanda C, Pego JM, et al. Transvesical endoscopic peritoneoscopy: a novel 5mm port for intra-abdominal scarless surgery. J Urol 2006;176:802–5.

37. Desai MM, Aron M, Berger A, et al. Transvesical robotic radical prostatectomy. BJU Int 2008;102:1666–9.

38. Pai RD, Fong DG, Bundga ME, et al. Transcolonic endoscopic cholecystectomy: a NOTES survival study in a porcine model (with video). Gastrointest Endosc 2006;64: 428–34.

39. Box GN, Lee HJ, Santos RJ, et al. Rapid communication: robot-assisted NOTES nephrectomy: initial report. J Endourol 2008;22:503–8.

40. Kaouk JH, Haber GP, Goel RK, et al. Single-port laparoscopic surgery in urology: initial experience. Urology 2008;71:3–6.

41. Kaouk JH, Goel RK, Haber GP, et al. Single-port laparoscopic radical prostatectomy. Urology 2008;72:1190–3.

42. Kaouk JH, Palmer JS. Single-port laparoscopic surgery: initial experience in children for varicocoelectomy. BJU Int 2008;102:97–9.

43. Haber GP, Crouzet S, Kamoi K, et al. Robotic NOTES (natural orifice transluminal endoscopic surgery) in reconstructive urology: initial laboratory experience. Urology 2008;71:996–1000.

44. Kaouk JH, Goel RK, Haber GP, et al. Robotic single-port transumbilical surgery in humans: initial report. BJU Int 2009;103:366–9.

45. Aron M, Canes D, Desai MM, et al. Transumbilical single port laparoscopic partial nephrectomy. BJU Int 2009;103:516–21.

46. Desai MM, Rao PP, Aron M, et al. Scarless single port transumbilical nephrectomy and pyeloplasty: first clinical report. BJU Int 2008;83:101–88.

47. Gill IS, Canes D, Aron M, et al. Single port transumbilical (E-NOTES) donor nephrectomy. J Urol 2008;180:637–41.

48. Canes D, Desai MM, Aron M, et al. Transumbilical single-port surgery: evolution and current status. Eur Urol 2008;54:1020–9.

49. Abbott DJ, Becke C, Rothstein RI, et al. Design of an endoluminal NOTES robotic system. Proceedings of 2007 IEEE/RSJ International Conference on Intelligent Robots and systems. San Diego, CA, October 29–November 2, 2007. p. 410–6.

50. Aron M, Haber GP, Desai MM, et al. Flexible robotics: a new paradigm. Curr Opin Urol 2007;17:151–5.

51. Desai MM, Aron M, Gill IS, et al. Flexible retrograde renoscopy: description of novel robotic device and preliminary laboratory experience. Urology 2008;72:42–6.

52. Okamura AM. Haptic feedback in robot-assisted minimally invasive surgery. Curr Opin Urol 2009;19:102–7.

53. Mahvash M. Novel approach for modeling separating forces between deformable bodies. IEEE Trans Inf Technol Biomed 2006;10:618–26.

54. Mahvash M, Hayward V. High fidelity haptic synthesis of contact with deformable bodies. IEEE Comput Graph Appl 2004;24:48–55.

55. Mahvash M, Voo LM, Kim D, et al. Modeling the forces of cutting with scissors. IEEE Trans Biomed Eng 2008;55:848–56.

56. Weiss H, Ortmaier T, Maass H, et al. A virtual reality based haptic surgical training system. Comput Aided Surg 2003;8:269–72.

57. Wagner CR, Howe RD. Force feedback benefit depends on experience in multiple degree of freedom robotic surgery. IEEE Trans Robot 2007;23:1235–40.

58. Rizun P, Gunn D, Cox B, et al. Mechatronic design for haptic forceps for robotic surgery. Int J Med Robot 2006;2:341–9.

59. Jurmain JC, Blancero AJ, Geiling JA, et al. Hazbot: development of a telemanipulator robot with haptics for emergency response. Am J Disaster Med 2008;3:87–97.

60. Available at: http://www.mimic.ws/products/MIMIC-dV-Trainer-Brochure.pdf. Accessed June 1, 2011.

61. Sweet RM, McDougall EM. Simulation and computer-animated devices: the new minimally invasive skills training paradigm. Urol Clin North Am 2008;35:519–31.

62. Lendvay TS, Casale P, Sweet R, et al. Initial validation of a virtual-reality robotic simulator. Journal of Robotic Surgery 2008;2:145–9.

63. Katsavelis D, Siu KC, Brown-Clerk B, et al. Validated robotic laparoscopic surgical training in a virtual-reality environment. Surg Endosc 2009;23:66–73.

64. Brown-Clerk B, Siu KC, Katsavelis D, et al. Validating advanced robotic-assisted laparoscopic training task in virtual reality. Stud Health Technol Inform 2008;132:45–9.

65. Available at: http://www.meti.com/products_ss_rss.htm. Accessed June 1, 2011.

66. Marescaux J, Leroy J, Gagner M, et al. Transatlantic robot-assisted telesurgery. Nature 2001;413:379–80.

67. Anvari M, McKinley C, Stein H. Establishment of the world's first telerobotic remote surgical service: for provision of advanced laparoscopic surgery in a rural community. Ann Surg 2005;241:460–4.

68. Sterbis JR, Hanly EJ, Herman BC, et al. Transcontinental telesurgical nephrectomy using the da Vinci robot in a porcine model. Urology 2008;71:971–3.

69. Lum MJH, Rosen J, King H, Telesurgery via unmanned aerial vehicle (UAV) with a field deployable surgical robot. In: Proceedings of Medicine Meets Virtual Reality (MMVR15). Long Beach, CA, 2007. p. 313–5

70. Bell CJ, Shenoy P, Chaladhorn R, et al. Control of a humanoid robot by a non-invasive brain-computer interface in humans. J Neural Eng 2008;5:214–20.

Robotic Surgery of the Mediastinum

Annemarie Weissenbacher, MD[a], Florian Augustin, MD[a],
Johannes Bodner, MD, MSc, FETCS[b],*

KEYWORDS

- Thoracic surgery • Robotics
- Video-assisted thoracoscopic surgery
- da Vinci robotic system • Mediastinum

Approximately 25 years ago, in the late 1980s, the revolutionary era of minimally invasive video-assisted surgery began. Initially introduced for abdominal surgery, it was soon adopted for thoracic procedures, and called video-assisted thoracoscopic surgery (VATS). Early procedures were technically simple like pleural biopsies or pleurodesis for persistent pleural effusion. However, technical progress and increased experience led to rapid expansion of indications to a variety of mediastinal and pulmonary procedures.[1]

Despite the well-proved benefits regarding patient recovery and cosmetics,[2,3] VATS has encountered significant drawbacks. For technically more advanced operations, especially oncologic procedures, the VATS approach is still limited to specific centers, and has not gained general acceptance and gold standard status. The two-dimensional visualization of the operative field, limited maneuverability of the thoracoscopic instruments, and bad ergonomics make VATS procedures, at least at the beginning, technically more challenging and may suggest reduced surgical accuracy and oncologic safety.[4]

To overcome these limitations, micromechanic and robotic technology was introduced in minimally invasive surgery in the mid-1990s.[5] When operating with the da Vinci surgical system, the surgeon sits at a console distant from the patient and triggers highly sensitive motion sensors that transfer the surgeon's movements to the tip of the instruments, which are attached to the arms of a surgical arm cart next to the patient.

An early critical evaluation of the potential, benefits, and disadvantages of robotic surgery revealed coronary artery bypass surgery[6,7] and prostatectomy[8,9] as domains

A version of this article was previously published in *Thoracic Surgery Clinics* 20:2.
[a] Department of Visceral, Transplant and Thoracic Surgery, Innsbruck Medical University, Anichstrasse 35, A-6020 Innsbruck, Austria
[b] Department of General, Visceral, Thoracic, Transplant and Pediatric Surgery, University Hospital Giessen, Marburg, Giessen, Germany
* Corresponding author.
E-mail address: Johannes.bodner@chiru.med.uni-giessen.de

for this new surgical approach. Because the technical benefits have most advantage in narrowly confined and difficult-to-reach anatomic regions, thoracic surgeons' interest soon focused on the mediastinum.[10]

MATERIALS AND METHODS
Anatomy of the Mediastinum

The mediastinum is the central department of the thoracic cavity, extending from the sternum in front to the vertebral column behind; it contains all the thoracic viscera except the lungs.

For the purpose of description, the mediastinum is divided into 2 parts:

1. The upper mediastinum is bounded by the thoracic inlet and the plane from the sternal angle to the disc of T4 to T5
2. The lower mediastinum can be subdivided into 3 parts
   - anterior mediastinum in front of the pericardium
   - middle mediastinum containing the pericardium and its contents
   - posterior mediastinum behind the pericardium.

Surgery of the Mediastinum

Diseases of the thymus, the esophagus, and the lymphatic tissue are the main indications for surgery of the mediastinum, and, more rarely, ectopic thyroid and parathyroid glands. A variety of benign as well as primary and secondary (metastatic) malignant lesions indicate surgical biopsy or resection (**Table 1**). Although in open surgery the mediastinum is approached either transcervically or via a sternotomy, for most minimally invasive video-assisted procedures the approach is transthoracic with incision of the mediastinal pleura.

Technical Aspects

The da Vinci system allows the surgeon to maintain the skills and techniques known from open surgery. The surgeon's intuitive hand movements are transferred from the console to inside the patient. Thus, any kind of mediastinal procedure performed with the robot is similar to the corresponding open operation. Robotic pick-ups are used for tissue grasping, a cautery hook or scissors are used for dissection, a robotic needle holder for

Table 1 Surgically relevant diseases of the mediastinum and corresponding minimally invasive procedures	
Disease	**Procedure**
Thymoma, thymic cyst, myasthenia gravis	(Extended) thym(mom)ectomy
(Paravertebral) neurinoma	Extirpation
Lymph node metastasis	Biopsy, sampling, oncologic dissection
Foregut cyst	Extirpation
Esophageal leiomyoma	Extirpation
Esophageal cancer	Dissection, resection, reconstruction
(Ectopic) parathyroid tissue	Extirpation
(Ectopic) thyroid tissue	Extirpation
Lymphoma	Biopsy (extirpation)
Germ cell tumors including teratoma	Extirpation

suturing. Control of major vessels is achieved either by direct ligation, by stitch tying, or with a robotic clip applier. Alternatively, conventional stapler devices can be introduced by the table-side assistant through an auxiliary port or, after intermittently removing 1 of the robotic instrument ports, through 1 of the initial incisions.

In robotic surgery, patient positioning, the placement of the robotic arm cart, and the positioning of the robotic and any eventual auxiliary trocars are crucial and procedure-specific. Poorly placed ports may cause collision of the robotic arms and thus hinder a successful operation.

Thymectomy and Thymomectomy

Robotic thymectomy has been performed from right-sided, left-sided, and bilateral approaches.[10–13] For any approach, patient positioning is incomplete (30–45°) lateral decubitus, with the approached side up; for a bilateral procedure the patient gets repositioned in the middle of the procedure.

A common position for the 0° or 30° camera is the fifth intercostal space in the midaxillary line.[10,12] Alternatively, the camera port is placed in the fourth intercostal space, anterior axillary line.[14] The robotic instrument ports are positioned in the third intercostal space, anterior to the midaxillary line, and in the fifth intercostal space, midclavicular line.[12,14] For best cosmetic results, especially in women, all 3 trocars are preferentially placed exactly along the submammary fold.[10] If necessary, auxiliary ports are introduced.[10,15,16]

The active lifting of the camera port (thoracolift)[15,16] and insufflation of CO_2 gas (6–10 mm Hg)[11] help to enlarge the space in the operative field, which improves visibility and instruments maneuverability.

An extended thymectomy with en bloc resection of the anterior mediastinal fat tissue following the rules of Masaoka and colleagues[17] is performed. The adipose tissue around the upper poles of the thymus, around both brachiocephalic veins, and on the pericardium is dissected meticulously. The resection borders are the diaphragm caudally, the thyroid gland cranially, and the phrenic nerves laterally on both sides. Smaller vessels are usually controlled by electrocautery, larger ones are ligated or clipped.[15,16]

Excision of Posterior Mediastinal Masses

Patient positioning varies from lateral decubitus[18] to supine.[19,20] Port placement depends on the position of the lesion with the camera port usually placed in the anterior axillary line, and the robotic instrument ports slightly anterior to the camera port.[19,20] For the resection of a paravertebral lesion, several auxiliary ports may be necessary.[21]

Dissection is performed with the cautery hook, usually without the need for ligation or clipping of any vessels.

Biopsy and Dissection of Mediastinal Lymph Nodes

In a minimally invasive esophagectomy for esophageal cancer, oncologic lymph node dissection is performed en bloc with the dissection of the thoracic esophagus.[22,23] Patient positioning is left lateral decubitus and the robot is placed dorsocranially. The 10-mm camera port is placed at the sixth intercostal space, posterior to the posterior axillary line. Two ports are placed anteriorly to the scapular rim in the fourth intercostal space and more posteriorly in the eighth intercostal space. Auxiliary thoracoscopic ports are used in the fifth and seventh intercostal spaces for assistance function. The lymph nodes from the subcarinal space (ATS7), the lower and middle paraesophageal

(ATS8) lymph nodes, the nodes within the inferior pulmonary ligament (ATS9), and the paratracheal lymph nodes (ATS2,4R) are dissected with the cautery hook or a robotic harmonic scalpel. Insufflating CO_2 to 10 mm Hg of pressure helps to evacuate cautery smoke and to compress the lung away from the operative area.[11,22]

Robotic lymph node dissection as part of an oncologic pulmonary lobectomy is essentially technically the same,[24] as is diagnostic biopsy of enlarged mediastinal lymph nodes in lymphoma patients. Patient positioning and port placement depend on the exact location of the lesion. A scapular roll can be used to elevate the appropriate side of the chest.[25]

Excision of Foregut Cyst

Foregut cysts are typically located in the lower esophagus in the posterior phrenico-costal sinus and may be partially covered by the esophageal muscular layer. The robotic trocars are placed anteriorly between the midclavicular and the midaxillary line. For better exposure, the diaphragm is intermittently fixed to the thoracic wall and the pulmonary ligament is divided with the cautery hook. The cyst is removed in an endobag.[26]

Excision of Esophageal Leiomyoma

Patient positioning for robotic extirpation of an esophageal leiomyoma is (in)complete left lateral decubitus position.[24,27] Typical port positions are the sixth intercostal space posterior to the posterior axillary line for the camera and the fourth and eighth intercostal spaces for the instruments. Two auxiliary ports in the fifth and seventh intercostal spaces for suction and retraction facilitate dissection. Esophageal myotomy and enucleation of the tumor are performed bluntly and with the robotic cautery hook.

Esophagectomy for Cancer

Patient positioning for robotic dissection of the thoracic esophagus as part of a (minimally invasive or open) 3-hole esophagectomy is (overwound) left lateral decubitus.[22-24] The esophagus is circumferentially mobilized with en bloc dissection of mediastinal lymph nodes.

For transhiatal esophagectomy patients are positioned in the semilithotomy position.[28] The robot is approached from the patient's head. Dissection of the esophagus is started at the hiatus and continued in a cephalad direction.

Excision of Ectopic Parathyroid Tissue

Depending on the exact location of the lesion a right-sided or left-sided approach is chosen. Patient positioning is (in)complete lateral decubitus. The camera port is situated in the fifth/sixth intercostal space in the anterior axillary line and the 2 instrument ports are placed 1 hand breadth right and left. The lung is retracted through an auxiliary port in the midclavicular line of the sixth intercostal space. Suction is provided via a second auxiliary port, positioned more posteriorly. Enucleation starts with the incision of the mediastinal pleura covering the aortopulmonary window. Caution has to be taken to avoid injury to the vagus and recurrent laryngeal nerves. The tumor is cautiously excised using blunt dissection and the cautery hook. The vascular pedicle is controlled with clips.[16,29,30]

Excision of Germ Cell Tumors

For resection of germ cell tumors and teratomas in the anterior mediastinum, patients are placed in a lateral decubitus position. The robot cart is positioned anteriorly.[31]

RESULTS

A systematic review of the literature revealed 24 papers reporting on a total of 257 patients who underwent minimally invasive surgery with the da Vinci robot in the mediastinum **(Table 2)**. The largest series are from Rueckert and colleagues (University Hospital Charité, Berlin, Germany)[14] who performed 95 extended thymectomies and from Bodner and colleagues and Augustin and colleagues[15,16,26] (Innsbruck University Hospital, Innsbruck, Austria) who reported on 5 different mediastinal procedures in a total of 49 patients. Overall, (extended) thymectomy is the by far most frequently performed procedure, representing 69.65% of all interventions. The second most common are esophageal procedures (esophagectomy, extirpation of leiomyoma) (21.40%). However, most of these operations were hybrid procedures in which the robot was used for some steps (dissection of the intrathoracic esophagus with en bloc lymph node dissection) only. Smaller series and single case reports deal with resections of posterior mediastinal paravertebral lesions and ectopic (para)thyroids.

Overall 253 (98.44%) procedures were successfully completed with the robot. From the 4 (1.56%) conversions to an open approach, 1 (0.39%) was an emergency conversion because of major bleeding. The overall intraoperative and postoperative complication rate was 1.56% and 20.23%, respectively. The 30-day mortality rate was 0.78%.

DISCUSSION

Robotic surgery was introduced almost 15 years ago.[32] Initial reports of the few general, cardiac, and thoracic surgeons who had early access to this new technique were characterized by great enthusiasm and the strong feeling that this was the beginning of a new surgical era.[5,33,34] An early and broad spread was predicted.

However, unlike the introduction of conventional laparoscopy and thoracoscopy, the surgical community appeared reluctant to become convinced. Was it just the high costs of the robot, making it an elitist device that was adored by those who had access to it but disdained by the broad majority who did not? Or have robotic surgery and robotic surgeons failed to furnish proof of a substantial benefit over conventional minimally invasive surgery?

Which procedures cannot be performed minimally invasively except when using the robot? After which procedures are the oncologic or functional results significantly better when performed with the robot? Positive answers to these questions would justify extra costs and rapidly and efficiently convince surgeons, patients, and health care providers.

So far the gold standard approach for the mediastinum is still open surgery. The mediastinum is a delicate and difficult to reach anatomic area. Working thoracoscopically in close proximity to vulnerable large vessels and nerves poses an increased risk. There is very little space, the image of the operating field on the monitor is two-dimensional only and a surgeon's tremor is heightened by the long instruments. Of any thoracic surgery, mediastinal procedures is the one for which the robot's characteristics have a significant advantage.

This review of all published papers reporting on robotic surgery of the mediastinum proves the feasibility and safety of a variety of procedures. For extended thymectomy, especially in patients suffering from myasthenia gravis, early and mid-term results suggest a benefit in the outcome when retrospectively compared with a conventional thoracoscopic or with an open approach.[10,12,14–16] Prospective randomized trials have been initiated to provide stronger evidence. Even if the results after robotic

Table 2
Summary of the literature on patients who underwent minimally invasive surgery with the da Vinci robot in the mediastinum (n = 257)

Main Author,[Ref] Year of Publication	Procedures (n)	Diagnosis	Results
Rueckert JC,[14] 2008	Extended thymectomy (95)	Myasthenia gravis	0 intraoperative complications 2 postoperative complications 1 conversion (advanced stage thymoma) 0% perioperative mortality Mean hospital stay: no data
Bodner J,[15,16,24,26] 2004, 2005, 2006	(Extended) thymectomy (32) Esophagectomy (5), robotic dissection of thoracic esophagus in Ivor-Lewis-esophagectomy Extirpation (2) Resection of (posterior) mediastinal mass (7) Lymph node dissection (1) Resection of mediastinal lesion (2)	Different thymic pathologies Esophageal cancer, esophageal leiomyoma Ectopic parathyroid, ectopic thyroid Neurinoma, lymphoma, ectopic Cushing, carcinoid Lymph node metastases Foregut cyst, traction diverticulum	0 intraoperative complications 2 postoperative complications 2 conversions (tumor size, malignancy) 0% perioperative mortality Mean hospital stay: 10 d
Rea F,[12] 2006	(Extended) thymectomy (33)	Myasthenia gravis	0 intraoperative complications 0 postoperative complications 0 conversion 0% perioperative mortality Mean hospital stay: 2.6 d
van Hillegersberg R,[23] 2006	Esophagectomy (21): robotic dissection of thoracic esophagus in 3-hole esophagectomy (conventional laparoscopic abdominal part)	Adenocarcinoma Squamous cell carcinoma	1 intraoperative complication (bleeding) 27 postoperative complications 1 conversion (bleeding) 4.6% perioperative mortality (1 patient) Mean hospital stay: 18 d

(continued on next page)

Table 2
(continued)

Main Author,[Ref] Year of Publication	Procedures (n)	Diagnosis	Results
Galvani CA,[28] 2008	Transhiatal esophagectomy (18): robotic dissection of thoracic esophagus in open 3-hole esophagectomy	Barrett esophagus (high-grade dysplasia) Adenocarcinoma	0 intraoperative complications 17 postoperative complications 0 conversions 0% perioperative mortality Mean hospital stay: no data
Savitt MA,[10] 2005	(Extended) thymectomy (18)	Different thymic pathologies	0 intraoperative complications 0 postoperative complications 0 conversions 0% perioperative mortality Mean hospital stay: 4 d
Giulianotti PC,[36] 2003	Esophagectomy (5) Resection (2)	Esophageal carcinoma Esophageal diverticulum, esophageal leiomyoma	0 intraoperative complications 2 postoperative complications 0 conversions 14.29% perioperative mortality Mean hospital stay: no data
Meehan JJ,[31] 2008	Resection of mediastinal lesion (5)	Germ cell tumor, ganglioneuroma, necrosis, ganglioneuroblastoma, mature teratoma	0 intraoperative complications 0 postoperative complications 0 conversions 0% perioperative mortality Mean hospital stay: 1,4 d
Morgan JA,[19,20] 2003	Resection of posterior mediastinal mass (2)	Neurofibroma, schwannoma	0 intraoperative complications 0 postoperative complications 0 conversions 0% perioperative mortality Mean hospital stay: 2 d

(continued on next page)

Table 2 (continued)			
Main Author,[Ref] Year of Publication	Procedures (n)	Diagnosis	Results
Yoshino I,[13,18] 2001, 2002	Extirpation (1) (Extended) thymectomy (1)	Bronchogenic cyst Thymoma	0 intraoperative complications 0 postoperative complications 0 conversions 0% perioperative mortality Mean hospital stay: no data
Boone J,[27] 2008	Esophagectomy (1) Robotic dissection of thoracic esophagus in open 3-hole esophagectomy	Esophageal leiomyoma	0 intraoperative complications 0 postoperative complications 0 conversions 0% perioperative mortality Hospital stay: 12 d
Brunaud L,[30] 2008	Resection (1)	Primary hyperparathyroidism (adenoma)	0 intraoperative complications 0 postoperative complications 0 conversions 0% perioperative mortality Hospital stay: no data
DeRose JJ,[25] 2003	Extirpation (1)	Diffuse B-large cell lymphoma	0 intraoperative complications 0 postoperative complications 0 conversions 0% perioperative mortality Hospital stay: 18 h
DeUgarte DA,[37] 2008	Extirpation (1)	Esophageal leiomyoma	0 intraoperative complications 0 postoperative complications 0 conversions 0% perioperative mortality Hospital stay: 5 d

(continued on next page)

Table 2
(continued)

Main Author,[Ref] Year of Publication	Procedures (n)	Diagnosis	Results
Kernstine KH,[22] 2004	Robotic esophagectomy and lymph node dissection (1), complete robotic thoracic and abdominal phase in 3-hole esophagectomy	Esophageal adenocarcinoma T3 N0	0 intraoperative complications 0 postoperative complications 0 conversions 0% perioperative mortality Hospital stay: 9 d
Ruurda JP,[21] 2003	Extirpation of thoracic neurogenic tumor (1)	Ancient schwannoma	0 intraoperative complications 0 postoperative complications 0 conversions 0% perioperative mortality Hospital stay: no data
Timmermann GL,[29] 2008	Extirpation (1)	Ectopic parathyroid (hyperparathyroidism)	0 intraoperative complications 0 postoperative complications 0 conversion 0% perioperative mortality Hospital stay: <72 h

thymectomy were not better but equal to conventional VATS thymectomy, the advantage of a single-sided approach would favor the robotic technique. This is achieved by the active lifting of the robotic camera port, which augments the operative space and by the high maneuverability of the tips of the robotic instruments.[15,16] When performed by conventional VATS, complete resection of all the retrosternal tissue between both phrenic nerves nearly always requires a bilateral approach or additional subxiphoid or cervical incisions.[35]

Based on numbers, esophageal surgery seems to be another domain for the robotic approach. However, there is a broad inhomogeneity with regard to technical details and the particular application of the robot within the specific groups.[22–24,27,28,36,37] In the 2 largest published series of Hillegersberg and colleagues[23] and Galvani and colleagues[28] the robot was used only for dissection of the thoracic esophagus during 3-hole-esophagectomies. Only Kernstine and colleagues[22] performed the entire procedure (except the cervical part) with the robot. Although there are so far only 3 single case reports,[24,27,37] extirpation/enucleation of esophageal leiomyomas as well as foregut cysts[26] seem to be an ideal indication for a robotic approach. These procedures comprise delicate dissection, precise myotomy, and final closure of the esophageal muscle layer. The three-dimensional image of the operating field displayed on the robotic console, automatic tremor filtering, and the multiarticulated tips of the robotic instruments facilitate these steps significantly.[24]

Resection of ectopic (para)thyroids are rare surgical indications.[16,29,30] However, (partial) median sternotomy or thoracotomy has been the standard approach for glands displaced deep in the anterior mediastinum. A conventional VATS approach is technically challenging, especially when located within the aortopulmonary window, and has not yet been reported in the English literature. So far 3 robotic resections of ectopic (para)thyroids in the aortopulmonary window have been reported.[16,30] Although 1 patient suffered from a transient left laryngeal recurrent nerve palsy, the feasibility of these procedures represents an example where the application of the robotic technology has clearly expanded the borders of minimally invasive thoracic surgery.

A critical evaluation of any benefits or disadvantages is a precondition when a new surgical technique is being introduced. Despite the impressive potential of the da Vinci robotic system, in general thoracic surgery indications for completely robotic procedures are limited. However, this does not seem to be true for mediastinal procedures, where the available data strongly suggest a substantial benefit over conventional VATS.

SUMMARY

Several different mediastinal procedures for benign and malignant diseases have been proved to be feasible and safe when performed by a robotic minimally invasive approach. This article reviews the published data on robotic mediastinal surgery, focusing on technical aspects and perioperative outcomes. These are evaluated for differences and potential benefits over open and conventional minimally invasive techniques. Is there a need for the robot in the mediastinum? Is its application justified?

REFERENCES

1. Roviaro GC, Varoli F, Vergani C, et al. State of the art in thoracoscopic surgery. A personal experience of 2000 videothoracoscopic procedures and an overview of the literature. Surg Endosc 2002;16:881–92.

2. Nagahiro I, Andou A, Aoe M, et al. Pulmonary function, postoperative pain, and serum cytokine level after obectomy: a comparison of VATS and conventional procedure. Ann Thorac Surg 2001;72:362–5.
3. Forster R, Storck M, Schafer JR, et al. Thoracoscopy versus thoracotomy: a prospective comparison of trauma and quality of life. Langenbecks Arch Surg 2002;387:32–6.
4. Dieter RA, Kuzycz GB. Complications and contraindications of thoracoscopy. Int Surg 1997;82:232–9.
5. Schurr MO, Arezzo A, Buess GF. Robotics and systems technology for advanced endoscopic procedures: experiences in general surgery. Eur J Cardiothorac Surg 1999;16(Suppl 2):97–105.
6. Bonatti J, Schachner T, Bernecker O, et al. Robotic totally endoscopic coronary artery bypass: program development and learning curve issues. J Thorac Cardiovasc Surg 2004;127(2):504–10.
7. Bonaros N, Schachner T, Wiedemann D, et al. Quality of life improvement after robotically assisted coronary artery bypass grafting. Cardiology 2009;114(1):59–66.
8. Tewari A, Peabody J, Sarle R, et al. Technique of da Vinci robot-assisted anatomic radical prostatectomy. Urology 2002;60:569–72.
9. Murphy DG, Kerger M, Crowe H, et al. Operative details and oncological and functional outcome of robotic-assisted laparoscopic radical prostatectomy: 400 cases with a minimum of 12 months follow-up. Eur Urol 2009;55:1358–66.
10. Savitt MA, Gao G, Furnary AP, et al. Application of robotic-assisted techniques to the surgical evaluation and treatment of the anterior mediastinum. Ann Thorac Surg 2005;79:450–5.
11. Kernstine KH. Robotics in thoracic surgery. Am J Surg 2004;188:89–97.
12. Rea F, Marulli G, Bortolotti L, et al. Experience with the "da Vinci" robotic system for thymectomy in patients with myasthenia gravis: report of 33 cases. Ann Thorac Surg 2006;81:455–9.
13. Yoshino I, Hashizume M, Shimada M, et al. Thoracoscopic thymectomy with the da Vinci computer-enhanced surgical system. J Thorac Cardiovasc Surg 2001;122: 783–5.
14. Rueckert JC, Ismail M, Swierzy M, et al. Thoracoscopic thymectomy with the da Vinci robotic system for myasthenia gravis. Ann NY Acad Sci 2008;1132:329–35.
15. Bodner J, Wykypiel H, Greiner A, et al. Early experience with robot-assisted surgery for mediastinal masses. Ann Thorac Surg 2004;78:259–65.
16. Bodner J, Wykypiel H, Wetscher G, et al. First experiences with the da Vinci™ operating robot in thoracic surgery. Eur J Cardiothorac Surg 2004;25:844–51.
17. Masaoka A, Yamakawa Y, Niwa H, et al. Extended thymectomy for myasthenia gravis patients: a 20-year review. Ann Thorac Surg 1996;62:853–9.
18. Yoshino I, Hashizume M, Shimada M, et al. Video-assisted thoracoscopic extirpation of a posterior mediastinal mass using the da Vinci computer enhanced surgical system. Ann Thorac Surg 2002;74:1235–7.
19. Morgan JA, Ginsburg ME, Sonett JR, et al. Advanced thoracoscopic procedures are facilitated by computer-aided robotic technology. Eur J Cardiothorac Surg 2003;23: 883–7.
20. Morgan JA, Kohmoto T, Smith CR, et al. Endoscopic computer-enhanced mediastinal mass resection using robotic technology. Heart Surg Forum 2003;6(6):E164–6.
21. Ruurda JP, Hanlo PW, Hennipman A, et al. Robot-assisted thoracoscopic resection of a benign mediastinal neurogenic tumor: technical note. Neurosurgery 2003;52(2): 462–4.
22. Kernstine KH, DeArmond DT, Karimi M, et al. The robotic, 2-stage, 3-field esophagolymphadenectomy. J Thorac Cardiovasc Surg 2004;127:1847–9.

23. van Hillegersberg R, Boone J, Daaisma WA, et al. First experience with robot-assisted thoracoscopic esophagolymphadenectomy for esophageal cancer. Surg Endosc 2006;20:1435–9.
24. Bodner JC, Zitt M, Ott H, et al. Robotic-assisted thoracoscopic surgery (RATS) for benign and malignant esophageal tumors. Ann Thorac Surg 2005;80:1202–6.
25. DeRose JJ, Swistel DG, Safavi A, et al. Mediastinal mass evaluation using advanced robotic techniques. Ann Thorac Surg 2003;75:571–3.
26. Augustin F, Schmid T, Bodner J. The robotic approach for mediastinal lesions. Int J Med Robot Comput Assist Surg 2006;2:262–70.
27. Boone J, Draaisma WA, Schipper MEI, et al. Robot-assisted thoracoscopic esophagectomy for a giant upper esophageal leiomyoma. Dis Esophagus 2008;21:90–3.
28. Galvani CA, Gorodner MV, Moser F, et al. Robotically assisted laparoscopic transhiatal esophagectomy. Surg Endosc 2008;22:188–95.
29. Timmermann GL, Allard B, Lovrien F, et al. Hyperparathyroidism: robotic-assisted thoracoscopic resection of a supernumary anterior mediastinal parathyroid tumor. J Laparoendosc Adv Surg Tech A 2008;18(1):76–9.
30. Brunaud L, Ayav A, Bresler L, et al. Da Vinci robot-assisted thoracoscopy for primary hyperparathyroidism: a new application in endocrine surgery. J Chir (Paris) 2008; 145(2):165–7.
31. Meehan JJ, Sandler AD. Robotic resection of mediastinal masses in children. J Laparoendosc Adv Surg Tech A 2008;18(1):114–9.
32. Himpens J, Leman G, Cadiére GB. Telesurgical laparoscopic cholecystectomy [letter]. Surg Endosc 1998;12:1091.
33. CadiÈre GB, Himpens J, Germay O, et al. Feasibility of robotic laparoscopic surgery: 146 cases. World J Surg 2001;25:1467–77.
34. Rassweiler J, Binder J, Frede T. Robotic and telesurgery: will they change our future?. Curr Opin Urol 2001;11:309–20.
35. Augustin F, Schmid T, Sieb M, et al. Video-assisted thoracoscopic surgery versus robotic-assisted thoracoscopic surgery thymectomy. Ann Thorac Surg 2008;85(2): 768–71.
36. Giulianotti PC, Coratti A, Angelini M, et al. Robotica in general surgery. Personal experience in a large community hospital. Arch Surg 2003;138:777–84.
37. DeUgarte DA, Teitelbaum D, Hirschl RB, et al. Robotic extirpation of complex massive esophageal leiomyoma. J Laparoendosc Adv Surg Tech A 2008;18(2):286–9.

Laparoscopic Liver Resection—Current Update

Kevin Tri Nguyen, MD, PhD, David A. Geller, MD*

KEYWORDS

- Laparoscopic liver resection • Laparoscopic hepatic resection
- Liver cancer • HCC • Colorectal cancer metastases

Laparoscopic hepatic resection is an emerging option in the field of hepatic surgery. With almost 3000 laparoscopic hepatic resections reported in the literature for benign and malignant tumors, with a combined mortality of 0.3% and morbidity of 10.5%, there will be an increasing demand for minimally invasive liver surgery.[1] Multiple series have been published on laparoscopic liver resections; however, no randomized controlled trial has been reported that compares laparoscopic with open liver resection. Large series, meta-analyses, and reviews have thus far attested to the feasibility and safety of minimally invasive hepatic surgery for benign and malignant lesions.[2–17] The largest single-center experience was published by Koffron and colleagues[3] and describes various minimally invasive approaches to liver resection, including pure laparoscopic, hand-assisted laparoscopic, and laparoscopic-assisted open (hybrid) techniques. The choice of the minimally invasive approach should depend on surgeon experience, tumor size, location, and the extent of liver resection.

This article reviews the literature on reports comparing laparoscopic with hepatic resections. Special emphasis is on the cumulative world literature on laparoscopic liver surgery, the consensus meeting on laparoscopic liver resection, the learning curve on laparoscopic liver resection, laparoscopic major hepatectomies, short-term benefits after laparoscopic liver resection, and survival outcomes for laparoscopic liver resection of hepatocellular carcinoma (HCC) and colorectal liver metastasis. Finally, financial cost comparisons are evaluated to determine the cost advantages or disadvantages of the laparoscopic approach.

WORLD REVIEW

Since the first laparoscopic liver resection was reported in 1992, there has been an exponential increase in the number of reported laparoscopic liver resection, with more than 127 published articles, totaling almost 3000 reported cases of laparoscopic liver

A version of this article was previously published in Surgical Clinics 90:4.
Department of Surgery, Starzl Transplant Institute, UPMC Liver Cancer Center, University of Pittsburgh, 3459 Fifth Avenue, UPMC Montefiore, 7 South, Pittsburgh, PA 15213-2582, USA
* Corresponding author.
E-mail address: gellerda@upmc.edu

Perioperative Nursing Clinics 6 (2011) 303–314
doi:10.1016/j.cpen.2011.06.004
1556-7931/11/$ – see front matter © 2011 Published by Elsevier Inc.

periopnursing.theclinics.com

resection.[1] Half of the reported cases were performed for malignant lesions and 45% for benign lesions. In addition, laparoscopic live donor hepatectomy was performed in 1.7% of cases. Several variations of the minimally invasive approach have been described, with the most commonly performed variation the pure laparoscopic approach (75%), followed distantly by the hand-assisted approach (17%) and the hybrid approach (2%). A hybrid approach is when the operation is started laparoscopically to mobilize the liver and perform the initial hilar dissection. Then, the parenchymal transection is completed through a small open incision or slight extension of the hand port incision.[18] The conversion rate from a laparoscopic approach to an open procedure was 4.1%. The most common type of laparoscopic liver resection performed is a wedge resection or segmentectomy (45%), followed by left lateral sectionectomy (20%). Major anatomic hepatectomies are still less frequently performed: right hepatectomy (9%) and left hepatectomy (7%). Cumulative morbidity and mortality was 10.5% and 0.3%.

INTERNATIONAL CONFERENCE ON LAPAROSCOPIC LIVER SURGERY

The first consensus meeting on laparoscopic liver surgery was held at the University of Louisville in Louisville, Kentucky, in November 2008, incorporating the opinions of the world's experts in laparoscopic and open liver surgery. The conference consisted of more than 125 liver surgeons from more than a dozen countries with 25 invited faculty members. From this meeting, consensus statements on laparoscopic liver surgery were formulated[19]:

1. Three terms should be used to describe laparoscopic liver resection: pure laparoscopy, hand-assisted laparoscopy, and the hybrid technique.
2. As in open hepatic resection, several different technical approaches for performing major laparoscopic liver resection have evolved. Similar to open liver surgery, no single method of parenchymal transection has been shown superior.
3. Major laparoscopic liver resections have been performed with safety and efficacy equal to that of open surgery in highly specialized centers.
4. The best indications for laparoscopic liver resection are in patients with solitary lesions, 5 cm or less, located in peripheral liver segments (segments 2–6). Major liver resections should be reserved for experienced surgeons already facile with more limited laparoscopic resections.
5. Conversion to an open liver resection should be performed for lack of case progression or patient safety.
6. Indications for surgery for benign hepatic lesions should not be expanded.
7. Resection (laparoscopic or open) remains the gold standard for the treatment of colorectal liver metastases.
8. When local resection for HCC is undertaken, it should be an anatomic segmental resection because this is associated with reduced local recurrence.
9. Laparoscopic live-donor hepatectomy remains the most controversial application of laparoscopic liver surgery and should only proceed in the confines of a worldwide registry.
10. A prospective randomized trial may be impractical due to difficulties defining the relevant study questions, the size of the study population, and the length of time to perform the trial. A cooperative patient registry may be more practical to help understand the role and safety of laparoscopic liver surgery.

THE LEARNING CURVE OF LAPAROSCOPIC LIVER RESECTION

Successful laparoscopic liver surgery requires expertise in advance laparoscopy and hepatobiliary surgery. An unknown number of cases, however, need to be performed to surpass the initial learning curve. The learning curve effect has been described for laparoscopic colorectal surgery and hernia repairs,[20–25] but until recently, no such study had been described for laparoscopic liver resection. Vigano and colleagues[26] evaluated the learning curve of laparoscopic liver resection. After adjusting for case-mix and potential confounders using the cumulative sum analysis, they showed that the learning curve for laparoscopic minor hepatectomies could be overcome with 60 cases. They showed that over 3 time periods in a 12-year span (1996–1999, 2000–2003, and 2004–2008), they performed a higher proportion of laparoscopic cases (17.5%, 22.4%, and 24.2%), laparoscopic resection for HCC (17.6%, 25.6, and 39.4%), laparoscopic resection of colorectal liver metastasis (0%, 6.4%, and 13%), and major hepatectomies (1.1%, 9.1%, and 8.5%). In addition, intraoperative outcomes were improved over time with less operative time (210, 180, and 150 minutes), less blood loss (300, 200, and 200 mL), and less conversion to open rate (15.5%, 10.3%, and 3.4%). Likewise, the Northwestern University group reported an increase in the percentage of total liver cases performed laparoscopically from 10% in 2002 to 80% in 2007.[3]

LAPAROSCOPIC MAJOR HEPATECTOMY

In the reported world literature, approximately 75% of cases performed were wedge resections, segmentectomies, or bisegmentectomies; however, 16% were anatomic hemihepatectomies.[1] The first reported major hepatectomies were reported by Hüscher and colleagues.[27] Widespread dissemination of laparoscopic major hepatectomies has been hindered by fears of major hemorrhage and the technical challenges of portal, caval, and hepatic vein dissection. Recently, Dagher and colleagues[28] reported an international, prospective study on 210 laparoscopic major liver resections (136 right and 74 left hepatectomies) in 5 medical centers (3 European, 2 United States, and 1 Australian) from 1997 to 2008. They showed an increasing number of laparoscopic major liver resections were performed each year. A pure laparoscopic approach was used in 43.3% of cases whereas a hand-assisted approach was used in 56.7% of cases. Conversion to laparotomy was required in 12.4% of cases. Mortality occurred in 1% of patients, and specific morbidity (hemorrhage, ascites, or biloma) occurred in 8.1% of patients. For patients with malignant disease, negative margins (R0 resections) were achieved in 97.4% of patients. Comparing the early experience (n = 90) with the late experience (n = 120), operative time, blood loss, portal clamping time, conversion rate, and hospital length of stay were improved over time. The investigators concluded from this multi-center, international study that laparoscopic major hepatectomy was feasible in selected patients, performed by surgeons already advanced in laparoscopic minor hepatectomies.

HEPATOCELLULAR CARCINOMA

HCC is the most common primary liver cancer worldwide with risk factors that include long-term excessive alcohol consumption, hepatitis B virus infection, hepatitis C virus infection, and metabolic liver diseases. For eligible patients, liver transplantation offers the highest recurrence-free survival rate; however, liver transplantation is limited due to a worldwide shortage of organs. For patents who do not meet transplantation criteria, liver resection offers the next best survival rate.

In the world literature, HCCs accounted for 52% of laparoscopic liver resections for malignant lesions.[1] Several studies have provided outcomes of laparoscopic resection for HCC (**Table 1**). Belli and colleagues[29] provide the largest matched comparison of laparoscopic (n = 54) with open liver resection (n = 125) of HCC in patients with cirrhosis. Mortalities at 30 days were similar between the two groups;

Table 1
Overall survival after laparoscopic liver resection for HCC studies

Authors	Year	No. of Patients	OS 1 Year (%)	OS 2 Years (%)	OS 3 Years (%)	OS 4 Years (%)	OS 5 Years (%)
Belli et al[29]	2009	54	—	—	67	—	—
Lai et al[30]	2009	30	—	—	—	—	50
Santambrogio et al[31]	2009	22	—	—	—	50	—
Sasaki et al[32]	2009	37	90	—	73	—	53
Cai et al[33]	2008	24	95.5	—	67.5	—	56.2
Chen et al[14]	2008	116	94.7	—	74.2	—	61.7
Dagher et al[34]	2008	32	—	—	71.9	—	—
Belli et al[35]	2007	23	—	86.9	—	—	—
Cherqui et al[36]	2006	27	—	—	93	—	—
Tang et al[37]	2006	17	86	59	—	—	—
Vibert et al[11]	2006	16	85	—	66	—	—
Kaneko et al[38]	2005	30	—	—	—	—	61
Teramoto et al[39]	2005	15	100	—	80	—	—
Laurent et al[40]	2003	13	—	—	89	—	—
Teramoto et al[41]	2003	11	—	—	—	—	75
Gigot et al[42]	2002	10	83.5	62.5	—	—	—
Shimada et al[43]	2001	17	85	—	70	—	50

Abbreviation: OS, overall survival.

however, morbidity was significantly lower in the laparoscopic group (19% vs 36%, $P = .02$). From an oncologic standpoint, the 3-year overall survival (67% vs 62%, $P = .347$) and disease-free survival (52% vs 59%, $P = .864$) between the laparoscopic and open groups were not significantly different. This important study supports the short-term benefits without the oncologic disadvantages of laparoscopic liver resection over open liver resection for HCC. These results are comparable with results of other studies showing an overall 3-year survival of 60% to 93% and 3-year disease-free survival of 52% to 64% after laparoscopic liver resection for HCC.[34,36,44]

Sarpel and colleagues[45] from the Mt Sinai group matched 20 laparoscopic liver resections for HCC to 56 open resections for HCC. Patients were well matched for age, gender, degree of cirrhosis, and tumor size. There were no significant differences in operative time or rates of blood transfusion whereas the laparoscopic patients had a shorter length of stay. There was no significant difference in positive margins or disease-free or overall survival between the groups. Five-year overall survival rates were also comparable in recent matched comparison studies of laparoscopic (50%–95%) with open (47%–75%) hepatic resection for HCC.[33,46,47]

Laparoscopic liver resection also facilitated subsequent liver transplantation after liver resection for HCC. Laurent and colleagues[48] performed 24 orthotopic liver transplants after prior liver resection for HCC (12 laparoscopic and 12 open liver resections). Indications for liver transplantation were recurrent HCC (n = 19) or planned bridge to transplant (n = 5). The same experienced liver transplant team performed the minimally invasive or open hepatic resection as well as subsequent liver transplantation. The laparoscopic group of patients had significantly fewer adhesions and facilitated the subsequent liver transplantation. Specifically, those patients who underwent prior laparoscopic liver resection had significantly less hepatectomy time (2.5 hours vs 4.5 hrs, $P<.05$), less total operating room time (6.2 hours vs 8.5 hours, $P<.05$), less blood loss (1.2 L vs 2.3 L, $P<.05$), and less blood transfusion (3 units vs 6 units packed red blood cells, $P<.05$) compared with the open group.

COLORECTAL CANCER LIVER METASTASIS

The new paradigm for surgical therapy of colorectal liver metastasis is resection, if possible, of all liver metastases with a negative margin while maintaining sufficient functional liver parenchyma with adequate inflow and outflow.[49] The standard approach to liver resection remains the open approach. The use of laparoscopy has, in the past, been limited to diagnostic laparoscopy to rule out extrahepatic disease that would preclude proceeding with open hepatic resection of the liver metastasis. Recent reports indicate that laparoscopic liver resection for colorectal liver metastasis is used in select patients with increasing frequency although not as often as laparoscopic hepatic resection for HCC (35% vs 52% of all reported laparoscopic liver resection for malignancy).[1] Major concerns about laparoscopic resection for colorectal cancer metastases include possible adhesions from prior intra-abdominal operation and the oncologic integrity of the resection. Data are emerging, however, to support minimally invasive hepatic resection for colorectal liver metastases. Nguyen and colleagues[2] reported a multi-institutional, international study on laparoscopic liver resection for metastatic colorectal cancer in 109 patients, 95% of whom had prior intra-abdominal operations. Oncologically, negative margins were achieved in 94.4% of patients and overall survivals at 1, 3, and 5 years were 88%, 69%, and 50% whereas disease-free survivals at 1, 3, and 5 years were 65%, 43%, and 43%. Other recent studies also report similar 5-year survival rates of 46% to 64% after laparoscopic liver resection of colorectal cancer metastases.[32,50] These 5-year survival results after laparoscopic liver resection of colorectal cancer metastases are comparable with overall 5-year survival results of 37% to 50% reported in modern open hepatic resection series from large liver cancer centers (**Table 2**). This study supports the safety and oncologic integrity of laparoscopic liver resection for colorectal cancer metastases in experienced centers.

The only head-to-head comparison of laparoscopic with open hepatectomy for colorectal liver metastases was performed by Castaing and colleagues.[51] They compared two groups (60 patients each) from two highly specialized liver surgery centers in France. From an oncologic standpoint, the laparoscopic approach was comparable with, if not better than, the open approach on several parameters. First, the laparoscopic group had a greater margin-free resection rate than the open group (87% vs 72%, $P = .04$). Second, the two groups had comparable overall survival, with 1-, 3-, and 5-year rates of 97%, 82%, and 64% in the laparoscopic group, and 97%, 70%, and 56% in the open group (log rank $P = .13$). Third, disease-free survival was comparable between the two groups with 1-, 3-, 5-year rates of 70%, 47%, and 35% in the laparoscopic group and 70%, 40%, and 27% in the open group (log rank $P = .32$). A limitation of this study is that the open hepatic resections were performed in a large volume hepatobiliary center, whereas the laparoscopic approach was performed by a single master minimally invasive surgery surgeon (BG). It is unclear whether or not these same results can be achieved on a broader scale. Nonetheless, the data support equivalent 5-year survival results of laparoscopic versus open hepatic resection for colorectal liver metastasis in selected patients.

BENEFITS OF LAPAROSCOPIC LIVER RESECTION

No prospective, randomized controlled trials have been established to compare laparoscopic with open liver resections. Several studies, however, have retrospectively compared laparoscopic with open liver resection. Many groups have shown decreased blood loss with laparoscopic versus open liver resection.[3,17,29,47,52,58–67] Postoperative pain control was better in laparoscopic cases with fewer days of required narcotic pain medication[52,68] and decreased total amount of pain medication required.[33,46,60,67,69,70]

More importantly, almost all the studies comparing laparoscopic with open liver resection consistently showed a significant earlier discharge to home after laparoscopic liver resection. Lengths of stay were variable based on the country of origin of the studies but were consistently shorter for laparoscopic liver resection. Three studies published in the United States[3,59,67] presented a length of stay of 1.9 to 4.0 days after laparoscopic liver resection. Studies from Europe[17,29,35,40,47,51,62–64,68,69,71–73] showed an average length of stay of 3.5 to 10 days whereas those from Asia[30,33,38,46,60,61,70] reported an average of length of stay of 4 to 20 days after laparoscopic liver resection.

COST ANALYSIS

There are concerns that the minimally invasive approach to liver resection may be associated with increased cost due to laparoscopic equipment/instrumentation. Koffron and colleagues[3] showed that the operating room costs for minimally invasive liver resections cases were significantly higher than those of open liver resection cases; however, these added expenses was more than offset by lower nonoperating room costs for the laparoscopic group, with the biggest factor a shorter length of stay. In their analysis, the operating room cost for right hemihepatectomy was 36% of total hospital costs for open cases compared with 47% of total hospital costs for minimally invasive cases; however, the nonoperating room costs were less with the minimally

Table 2
Laparoscopic versus open hepatic resection for colorectal cancer metastases

Authors (Laparoscopic)	Year	Journal	No. of Patients	OS 3 Years (%)	OS 5 Years (%)
Kazaryan et al[50]	2010	Arch Surg	96	79	46
Nguyen et al[2]	2009	Ann Surg	109	69	50
Castaing et al[51]	2009	Ann Surg	60	82	64
Sasaki et al[32]	2009	Br J Surg	39	64	64
Ito et al[52]	2009	J Gastrointest Surg	13	72	—
Robles et al[53]	2008	Surg Endosc	21	80	—
Vibert et al[11]	2006	Br J Surg	41	87	—
O'Rourke and Fielding[8]	2004	J Gastrointest Surg	22	75 (2 y)	—
Gigot et al[42]	2002	Ann Surg	27	100 (2 y)	—
Authors (Open)	**Year**	**Journal**	**No. of Patients**	**OS 3 Years (%)**	**OS 5 Years (%)**
Ito et al[54]	2008	Ann Surg	1067	65	45
Blazer et al[55]	2008	J Clin Oncol	305	65	42
Adam et al[56]	2008	J Clin Oncol	738	61	45
Zakaria et al[57]	2007	Ann Surg	662	55	37

Abbreviation: OS, overall survival.

invasive group. Specifically, the nonoperating room costs for right hemihepatectomy were 64% of total hospital costs for open cases compared with 35% of total hospital costs for minimally invasive cases. This cost differential was significantly dependent on length of hospital stay ($P<.0001$).[3] Rowe and colleagues[66] showed that the costs of stapler/trocar devices were similar between the laparoscopic and the open groups whereas Polignano and colleagues[64] showed that disposable instruments and other devices were significantly higher for laparoscopic hepatic resection versus open hepatic resection ($P<.0001$). Two studies confirmed, however, that overall hospital costs were less for the laparoscopic group due to shorter lengths of stay ($P\le.04$).[64,67] Vanounou and colleagues[74] used deviation-based cost modeling to compare the costs of laparoscopic with open left lateral sectionectomy at the University of Pittsburgh Medical Center. They compared 29 laparoscopic with 40 open cases and showed that patients who underwent the laparoscopic approach faired more favorably with a shorter length of stay (3 vs 5 days, $P<.0001$), significantly less postoperative morbidity ($P = .001$), and a weighted-average median cost savings of $1527 to $2939 per patient compared with patients who underwent open left lateral sectionectomy.

CANCER OUTCOMES
Surgical Margins

Initial concerns about the adequacy of surgical margins and possible tumor seeding prevented the widespread adoption of laparoscopic resection approaches for liver cancers. In comparison studies, there were no differences in margin-free resections between laparoscopic and open liver resection.[17,29,33,35,40,45–47,51,52,60,64–67,72] In addition, no incidence of port-site recurrence or tumor seeding has been reported. With more than 3000 cases of minimally invasive hepatic resection reported in the literature (and no documentation of any significant port-site or peritoneal seeding), the authors conclude that this concern should not prevent surgeons from accepting a laparoscopic approach.

Survival Outcomes

There were no significant differences in overall survival in the 13 studies that compared laparoscopic liver resection with open liver resection for cancer.[29,30,33,35,38,40,43,45–47,51,52,60] For example, Cai and colleagues[33] showed that the 1-, 3-, and 5-year survival rates after laparoscopic resection of HCC were 95.4%, 67.5%, and 56.2% versus 100%, 73.8%, and 53.8% for open resection. For resection of colorectal cancer liver metastasis, Ito and colleagues[52] showed a 3-year survival of 72% after laparoscopic liver resection and 56% after open liver resection whereas Castaing and colleagues[51] showed a 5-year survival of 64% after laparoscopic liver resection versus 56% after open liver resection.

DISCUSSION

Compared with open liver resections, laparoscopic liver resections are associated with less blood loss, less pain medication requirement, and shorter length of hospital stay. A randomized controlled clinical trial is the best method to compare laparoscopic with open liver resection; however, such a trial may be difficult to conduct because patients are unlikely to subject themselves to an open procedure when a minimally invasive approach has been shown feasible and safe in experienced hands. In addition, many patients would have to be accrued to detect a difference in complications that occur infrequently. Short of a large randomized clinical trial, meta-analysis and matched comparisons provide the next best option to compare laparoscopic with open liver resection.

For laparoscopic resection of HCC or colorectal cancer metastases, there has been no difference in 5-year overall survival compared with open hepatic resection. In addition, from a financial standpoint, the minimally invasive approach to liver resection may be associated with higher operating room costs; however, the total hospital costs were offset or improved due to the associated shorter length of hospital stay with the minimally invasive approach.

SUMMARY

Minimally invasive hepatic resection for benign and malignant liver lesions is safe and feasible with short-term benefits, no economic disadvantage, and no compromise to oncologic principles. These results indicate that laparoscopic hepatic resection is an important part of the armamentarium in hepatic resection surgery in selected patients.

REFERENCES

1. Nguyen KT, Gamblin TC, Geller DA. World review of laparoscopic liver resection—2,804 patients. Ann Surg 2009;250(5):831–41.
2. Nguyen KT, Laurent A, Dagher I, et al. Minimally invasive liver resection for metastatic colorectal cancer: a multi-institutional, international report of safety, feasibility, and early outcomes. Ann Surg 2009;250(5):842–8.
3. Koffron AJ, Auffenberg G, Kung R, et al. Evaluation of 300 minimally invasive liver resections at a single institution: less is more. Ann Surg 2007;246(3):385–92.
4. Koffron AJ, Geller DA, Gamblin TC, et al. Laparoscopic liver surgery: Shifting the management of liver tumors. Hepatology 2006;44(6):1694–700.
5. Gamblin TC, Holloway SE, Heckman JT, et al. Laparoscopic resection of benign hepatic cysts: a new standard. J Am Coll Surg 2008;207(5):731–6.
6. Buell JF, Thomas MT, Rudich S, et al. Experience with more than 500 minimally invasive hepatic procedures. Ann Surg 2008;248(3):475–86.
7. Descottes B, Glineur D, Lachachi F, et al. Laparoscopic liver resection of benign liver tumors. Surg Endosc 2003;17(1):23–30.
8. O'Rourke N, Fielding G. Laparoscopic right hepatectomy: surgical technique. J Gastrointest Surg 2004;8(2):213–6.
9. Are C, Fong Y, Geller DA. Laparoscopic liver resections. Adv Surg 2005;39:57–75.
10. Cai XJ, Yu H, Liang X, et al. Laparoscopic hepatectomy by curettage and aspiration. Experiences of 62 cases. Surg Endosc 2006;20(10):1531–5.
11. Vibert E, Perniceni T, Levard H, et al. Laparoscopic liver resection. Br J Surg 2006;93(1):67–72.
12. Dagher I, Proske JM, Carloni A, et al. Laparoscopic liver resection: results for 70 patients. Surg Endosc 2007;21(4):619–24.
13. Simillis C, Constantinides VA, Tekkis PP, et al. Laparoscopic versus open hepatic resections for benign and malignant neoplasms—a meta-analysis. Surgery 2007;141(2):203–11.
14. Chen HY, Juan CC, Ker CG. Laparoscopic liver surgery for patients with hepatocellular carcinoma. Ann Surg Oncol 2008;15(3):800–6.
15. Cho J, Han H, Yoon Y, et al. Experiences of laparoscopic liver resection including lesions in the posterosuperior segments of the liver. Surg Endosc 2008;22(11):2344–9.
16. Pulitanò C, Aldrighetti L. The current role of laparoscopic liver resection for the treatment of liver tumors. Nat Clin Pract Gastroenterol Hepatol 2008;5(11):648–54.

17. Topal B, Fieuws S, Aerts R, et al. Laparoscopic versus open liver resection of hepatic neoplasms: comparative analysis of short-term results. Surg Endosc 2008;22(10): 2208–13.
18. Koffron AJ, Kung RD, Auffenberg GB, et al. Laparoscopic liver surgery for everyone: the hybrid method. Surgery 2007;142(4):463–8.
19. Buell JF, Cherqui D, Geller DA, et al. The international position on laparoscopic liver surgery: the Louisville Statement, 2008. Ann Surg 2009;250(5):825–30.
20. Lal P, Kajla RK, Chander J, et al. Laparoscopic total extraperitoneal (TEP) inguinal hernia repair: overcoming the learning curve. Surg Endosc 2004;18(4):642–5.
21. Bencini L, Sánchez LJ. Learning curve for laparoscopic ventral hernia repair. Am J Surg 2004;187(3):378–82.
22. Haidenberg J, Kendrick ML, Meile T, et al. Totally extraperitoneal (TEP) approach for inguinal hernia: the favorable learning curve for trainees. Curr Surg 2003;60(1):65–8.
23. Edwards CC 2nd, Bailey RW. Laparoscopic hernia repair: the learning curve. Surg Laparosc Endosc Percutan Tech 2000;10(3):149–53.
24. Tekkis PP, Senagore AJ, Delaney CP, et al. Evaluation of the learning curve in laparoscopic colorectal surgery: comparison of right-sided and left-sided resections. Ann Surg 2005;242(1):83–91.
25. Schlachta CM, Mamazza J, Seshadri PA, et al. Defining a learning curve for laparoscopic colorectal resections. Dis Colon Rectum 2001;44(2):217–22.
26. Vigano L, Laurent A, Tayar C, et al. The learning curve in laparoscopic liver resection: improved feasibility and reproducibility. Ann Surg 2009;250(5):772–82.
27. Hüscher CG, Lirici MM, Chiodini S, et al. Current position of advanced laparoscopic surgery of the liver. J R Coll Surg Edinb 1997;42(4):219–25.
28. Dagher I, O'Rourke N, Geller DA, et al. Laparoscopic major hepatectomy: an evolution in standard of care. Ann Surg 2009;250(5):856–60.
29. Belli G, Limongelli P, Fantini C, et al. Laparoscopic and open treatment of hepatocellular carcinoma in patients with cirrhosis. Br J Surg 2009;96(9):1041–8.
30. Lai EC, Tang CN, Yang GP, et al. Minimally invasive surgical treatment of hepatocellular carcinoma: long-term outcome. World J Surg 2009;33(10):2150–4.
31. Santambrogio R, Aldrighetti L, Barabino M, et al. Laparoscopic liver resections for hepatocellular carcinoma. Is it a feasible option for patients with liver cirrhosis? Langenbecks Arch Surg 2009;394(2):255–64.
32. Sasaki A, Nitta H, Otsuka K, et al. Ten-year experience of totally laparoscopic liver resection in a single institution. Br J Surg 2009;96(3):274–9.
33. Cai XJ, Yang J, Yu H, et al. Clinical study of laparoscopic versus open hepatectomy for malignant liver tumors. Surg Endosc 2008;22(11):2350–6.
34. Dagher I, Lainas P, Carloni A, et al. Laparoscopic liver resection for hepatocellular carcinoma. Surg Endosc 2008;22(2):372–8.
35. Belli G, Fantini C, D'Agostino A, et al. Laparoscopic versus open liver resection for hepatocellular carcinoma in patients with histologically proven cirrhosis: short- and middle-term results. Surg Endosc 2007;21(11):2004–11.
36. Cherqui D, Laurent A, Tayar C, et al. Laparoscopic liver resection for peripheral hepatocellular carcinoma in patients with chronic liver disease: midterm results and perspectives. Ann Surg 2006;243(4):499–506.
37. Tang CN, Tsui KK, Ha JP, et al. A single-centre experience of 40 laparoscopic liver resections. Hong Kong Med J 2006;12(6):419–25.
38. Kaneko H, Takagi S, Otsuka Y, et al. Laparoscopic liver resection of hepatocellular carcinoma. Am J Surg 2005;189(2):190–4.

39. Teramoto K, Kawamura T, Takamatsu S, et al. Laparoscopic and thoracoscopic approaches for the treatment of hepatocellular carcinoma. Am J Surg 2005;189(4): 474–8.
40. Laurent A, Cherqui D, Lesurtel M, et al. Laparoscopic liver resection for subcapsular hepatocellular carcinoma complicating chronic liver disease. Arch Surg 2003;138(7): 763–9.
41. Teramoto K, Kawamura T, Takamatsu S, et al. Laparoscopic and thoracoscopic partial hepatectomy for hepatocellular carcinoma. World J Surg 2003;27(10):1131–6.
42. Gigot JF, Glineur D, Santiago Azagra J, et al. Laparoscopic liver resection for malignant liver tumors: preliminary results of a multicenter European study. Ann Surg 2002;236(1):90–7.
43. Shimada M, Hashizume M, Maehara S, et al. Laparoscopic hepatectomy for hepato-cellular carcinoma. Surg Endosc 2001;15(6):541–4.
44. Lai EC, Tang CN, Ha JP, et al. Laparoscopic liver resection for hepatocellular carcinoma: ten-year experience in a single center. Arch Surg 2009;144(2):143–7.
45. Sarpel U, Hefti MM, Wisnievsky JP, et al. Outcome for patients treated with laparo-scopic versus open resection of hepatocellular carcinoma: case-matched analysis. Ann Surg Oncol 2009;16(6):1572–7.
46. Endo Y, Ohta M, Sasaki A, et al. A comparative study of the long-term outcomes after laparoscopy-assisted and open left lateral hepatectomy for hepatocellular carcinoma. Surg Laparosc Endosc Percutan Tech 2009;19(5):e171–4.
47. Tranchart H, Di Giuro G, Lainas P, et al. Laparoscopic resection for hepatocellular carcinoma: a matched-pair comparative study. Surg Endosc 2010;24(5):1170–6.
48. Laurent A, Tayar C, Andréoletti M, et al. Laparoscopic liver resection facilitates salvage liver transplantation for hepatocellular carcinoma. J Hepatobiliary Pancreat Surg 2009;16(3):310–4.
49. Mayo SC, Pawlik TM. Current management of colorectal hepatic metastasis. Expert Rev Gastroenterol Hepatol 2009;3(2):131–44.
50. Kazaryan AM, Pavlik Marangos I, Rosseland AR, et al. Laparoscopic liver resection for malignant and benign lesions: ten-year Norwegian single-center experience. Arch Surg 2010;145(1):34–40.
51. Castaing D, Vibert E, Ricca L, et al. Oncologic results of laparoscopic versus open hepatectomy for colorectal liver metastases in two specialized centers. Ann Surg 2009;250(5):849–55.
52. Ito K, Ito H, Are C, et al. Laparoscopic versus open liver resection: a matched-pair case control study. J Gastrointest Surg 2009;13(12):2276–83.
53. Robles R, Marín C, Abellán B, et al. A new approach to hand-assisted laparoscopic liver surgery. Surg Endosc 2008;22(11):2357–64.
54. Ito H, Are C, Gonen M, et al. Effect of postoperative morbidity on long-term survival after hepatic resection for metastatic colorectal cancer. Ann Surg 2008;247(6):994–1002.
55. Blazer DG 3rd, Kishi Y, Maru DM, et al. Pathologic response to preoperative chemo-therapy: a new outcome end point after resection of hepatic colorectal metastases. J Clin Oncol 2008;26(33):5344–51.
56. Adam R, Wicherts DA, de Haas RJ, et al. Complete pathologic response after preoperative chemotherapy for colorectal liver metastases: myth or reality? J Clin Oncol 2008;26(10):1635–41.
57. Zakaria S, Donohue JH, Que FG, et al. Hepatic resection for colorectal metastases: value for risk scoring systems? Ann Surg 2007;246(2):183–91.
58. Lesurtel M, Cherqui D, Laurent A, et al. Laparoscopic versus open left lateral hepatic lobectomy: a case-control study. J Am Coll Surg 2003;196(2):236–42.

59. Buell JF, Thomas MJ, Doty TC, et al. An initial experience and evolution of laparoscopic hepatic resectional surgery. Surgery 2004;136(4):804–11.
60. Lee KF, Cheung YS, Chong CN, et al. Laparoscopic versus open hepatectomy for liver tumours: a case control study. Hong Kong Med J 2007;13(6):442–8.
61. Mamada Y, Yoshida H, Taniai N, et al. Usefulness of laparoscopic hepatectomy. J Nippon Med Sch 2007;74(2):158–62.
62. Abu Hilal M, McPhail MJ, Zeidan B, et al. Laparoscopic versus open left lateral hepatic sectionectomy: a comparative study. Eur J Surg Oncol 2008;34(12):1285–8.
63. Aldrighetti L, Pulitanò C, Catena M, et al. A prospective evaluation of laparoscopic versus open left lateral hepatic sectionectomy. J Gastrointest Surg 2008;12(3):457–62.
64. Polignano FM, Quyn AJ, de Figueiredo RS, et al. Laparoscopic versus open liver segmentectomy: prospective, case-matched, intention-to-treat analysis of clinical outcomes and cost effectiveness. Surg Endosc 2008;22(12):2564–70.
65. Dagher I, Di Giuro G, Dubrez J, et al. Laparoscopic versus open right hepatectomy: a comparative study. Am J Surg 2009;198(2):173–7.
66. Rowe AJ, Meneghetti AT, Schumacher PA, et al. Perioperative analysis of laparoscopic versus open liver resection. Surg Endosc 2009;23(6):1198–203.
67. Tsinberg M, Tellioglu G, Simpfendorfer CH, et al. Comparison of laparoscopic versus open liver tumor resection: a case-controlled study. Surg Endosc 2009;23(4):847–53.
68. Mala T, Edwin B, Gladhaug I, et al. A comparative study of the short-term outcome following open and laparoscopic liver resection of colorectal metastases. Surg Endosc 2002;16(7):1059–63.
69. Farges O, Jagot P, Kirstetter P, et al. Prospective assessment of the safety and benefit of laparoscopic liver resections. J Hepatobiliary Pancreat Surg 2002;9(2):242–8.
70. Tang CN, Tai CK, Ha JP, et al. Laparoscopy versus open left lateral segmentectomy for recurrent pyogenic cholangitis. Surg Endosc 2005;19(9):1232–6.
71. Rau HG, Buttler E, Meyer G, et al. Laparoscopic liver resection compared with conventional partial hepatectomy–a prospective analysis. Hepatogastroenterology 1998;45(24):2333–8.
72. Morino M, Morra I, Rosso E, et al. Laparoscopic vs open hepatic resection: a comparative study. Surg Endosc 2003;17(12):1914–8.
73. Troisi R, Montalti R, Smeets P, et al. The value of laparoscopic liver surgery for solid benign hepatic tumors. Surg Endosc 2008;22(1):38–44.
74. Vanounou T, Steel J, Nguyen KT, et al. Comparing the clinical and economic impact of laparoscopic versus open liver resection. Ann Surg Oncol 2010;17(4):998–1009.

Index

Note: Page numbers of article titles are in **boldface** type.

A

Acubot robots, 274
Advocacy, **235–240**
Anesthesia, 223, 244–246
Antibiotics, for prostatectomy, 244, 249
Anxiety, 236
Appendectomy, 285
Automated Endoscopic System for Optimal Positioning (AESOP), 27

B

Benner "Novice to Expert Theory," 202, 206
Biliary-enteric reconstruction, 263
Biopsy specimen retrieval, in prostatectomy, 249
Bowel injury, in renal surgery, 255–256

C

Cardiac arrest, in renal surgery, 255
Cholecystectomy, 278, 284
Colorectal cancer, metastatic, liver resection for, 307–308, 310
Colorectal resection, liver resection with, 263–264
Computer Motion systems, 214
Coordinator, for robotic surgery, 220–221, 228–229

D

da Vinci robots
  description of, 201–204, 214–217
  disadvantages of, 275
  for liver surgery, **259–272**
  for urologic surgery, **241–258**
  technologic advances in, **273–289**
  training for, 206–209
Drain placement, for prostatectomy, 249
Draping, 205
dV-Trainer, 283

E

Education and training (health care workers)
  documentation of, 209
  for common errors, 207–209

Perioperative Nursing Clinics 6 (2011) 315–320
doi:10.1016/S1556-7931(11)00043-X
1556-7931/11/$ – see front matter © 2011 Elsevier Inc. All rights reserved.

S

Printed and bound by CPI Group (UK) Ltd, Croydon, CR0 4YY

03/10/2024

01040450-0015